Online Psychoanalysis

Written in clear and accessible language, this book offers an engaging and timely exploration of how the digital revolution is reshaping psychodynamic practice.

Drawing on the latest research and clinical insights, Haim Weinberg examines the impact and effectiveness of online psychodynamic psychotherapy compared to in-person work. The book delves deeply into the therapeutic alliance – the factor most strongly linked to positive outcomes – and explores the unique challenges therapists face in virtual settings: Loss of control over the therapeutic environment, the disembodied nature of online encounters, and the struggle to maintain presence. For each obstacle, Weinberg provides practical, creative strategies, including methods for reading nonverbal cues, handling technical disruptions, and navigating transference and countertransference when technology becomes part of the analytic matrix. The text also covers multiple formats – individual, couple, and group therapy – and discusses how core psychodynamic processes are preserved and transformed online.

Online Psychoanalysis: A Contemporary Introduction is an essential resource for students, trainees, and experienced clinicians eager to understand and master the online therapeutic space.

Haim Weinberg is a psychologist, group analyst, and certified group psychotherapist based in Sacramento, CA. He has developed group therapy training groups in Asia, and leads online training process groups for therapists around the world.

Routledge Introductions to Contemporary Psychoanalysis

Series Editor: Aner Govrin
Executive Editor: Yael Peri Herzovich

Otto Kernberg: A Contemporary Introduction
Frank Yeomans, Diana Diamond, Eve Caligor

Erich Fromm: A Contemporary Introduction
Sandra Buechler

Narcissism: A Contemporary Introduction
Richard Wood

The Death Drive: A Contemporary Introduction
Rossella Valdrè

Depression: A Contemporary Introduction
Marianne Leuzinger-Bohleber

Ronald Fairbairn: A Contemporary Introduction
David P. Celani

The Evidence for Psychodynamic Psychotherapy: A Contemporary Introduction
Kevin McCarthy, Carla Capone and Liat Leibovich

Psychoanalytic Group Psychotherapy: A Contemporary Introduction
Richard M. Billow

"With the advent of digital communications technology we all now live in a vastly altered world. Never before has the practice and framework of psychotherapy changed so rapidly and universally and we are all trying to adapt and understand what this all means and how it affects our patients and our work. This book is the singularly most valuable book to help every clinician, of whatever persuasion, think through this new world. Haim Weinberg is the world's premier authority on online psychotherapy. Addressing the current state of online treatment, the most up-to-date research findings, how online treatment effects the therapeutic alliance, transference and countertransference, the impact on boundaries, confidentiality and privacy, and the unique considerations for couples and group treatment online, this book leaves no stone unturned and no question unanswered. Haim Weinberg guides us through this new and confusing terrain with clarity, wisdom, and common sense. This book is the essential guide to online psychotherapy right now."

Robert Grossmark, PhD, ABPP, *psychoanalyst in private practice in New York City. New York University Postdoctoral Program in Psychoanalysis and Psychotherapy. Author of* The Unobtrusive Relational Analyst: Explorations in Psychoanalytic Companioning

"Imagine a future where AI technologies allow us to be transported into the consulting room anywhere on the planet or beyond. Since the global pandemic, the world has gone virtual. Psychoanalysis is no exception. It must adapt in order to survive and thrive. In this concise introduction to the parameters, advantages, and liabilities of online therapy, Haim Weinberg convinces us that we must keep up with the times. Whether you are for or against it, he cogently lays out the pros and cons and easily establishes himself as the leading authority on the topic."

Prof. Jon Mills, PsyD, PhD, ABPP, *author of* End of the World: Civilization and Its Fate, *Honorary Professor, Department of Psychosocial & Psychoanalytic Studies, University of Essex,*

UK, Faculty, Postgraduate Programs in Psychoanalysis & Psychotherapy, Gordon F. Derner School of Psychology, Adelphi University, USA, Faculty, New School for Existential Psychoanalysis, USA

Existential Psychoanalysis: A Contemporary Introduction
M. Guy Thompson

Dreams and Dream Interpretation: A Contemporary Introduction
Christian Roesler

Interpersonal Psychoanalysis: A Contemporary Introduction
Anna Maria Loiacono

Psychodynamic and Psychoanalytic Supervision: A Contemporary Introduction
Christine Driver

Couple Relations: A Contemporary Introduction
Mary Morgan

The Oedipus Complex: A Contemporary Introduction
Poul Rohleder

Psychoanalytic Film Theory: A Contemporary Introduction
Ben Tyrer

Thomas Ogden: A Contemporary Introduction
Ofrit Shapira-Berman

Online Psychoanalysis: A Contemporary Introduction
Haim Weinberg

Psychosis: A Contemporary Introduction
Franco De Masi

For more information about this series, please visit: www.routledge.com/Routledge-Introductions-to-Contemporary-Psychoanalysis/book-series/ICP

Online Psychoanalysis

A Contemporary Introduction

Haim Weinberg

Routledge
Taylor & Francis Group
LONDON AND NEW YORK

Designed cover image: © Michal Heiman, Asylum 1855–2020, The Sleeper (video, psychoanalytic sofa and Plate 34), exhibition view, Herzliya Museum of Contemporary Art, 2017

First published 2026
by Routledge
4 Park Square, Milton Park, Abingdon, Oxon OX14 4RN

and by Routledge
605 Third Avenue, New York, NY 10158

Routledge is an imprint of the Taylor & Francis Group, an informa business

British Library Cataloguing-in-Publication Data
A catalogue record for this book is available from the British Library

ISBN: 978-1-032-82216-7 (hbk)
ISBN: 978-1-032-80661-7 (pbk)
ISBN: 978-1-003-50351-4 (ebk)

DOI: 10.4324/9781003503514

Typeset in Times New Roman
by Taylor & Francis Books

To my beloved wife, whose love, patience, and unwavering support have been my anchor through every challenge and inspiration in every endeavor.

To my children and grandchildren, who bring joy, meaning, and hope to my life, and remind me daily of the power of connection across generations.

And to my patients, past and present, whose courage, trust, and openness have been my greatest teachers – this book is, in many ways, a reflection of all you have taught me.

Contents

Series Editor's Preface

Aner Govrin

Routledge Introductions to Contemporary Psychoanalysis is one of the most prominent psychoanalytic publishing ventures of our day. The series' aim is to become an encyclopedia of psychoanalysis, with each entry given its own book.

This comprehensive series illuminates the intricate landscape of psychoanalytic theory and practice. In this collection of concise yet illuminating volumes, we delve into the influential figures, groundbreaking concepts, and transformative theories that shape the contemporary psychoanalytic landscape.

At the heart of each volume lies a commitment to clarity, accessibility, and depth. Our expert authors, renowned scholars and practitioners in their respective fields, guide readers through the complexities of psychoanalytic thought with precision and enthusiasm. Whether you are a seasoned psychoanalyst, a student eager to explore the field, or a curious reader seeking insight into the human psyche, our series offers a wealth of knowledge and insight.

Each volume serves as a gateway into a specific aspect of psychoanalytic theory and practice. From the pioneering works of Sigmund Freud to the innovative contributions of modern theorists such as Antonino Ferro and Michal Eigen, our series covers a diverse range of topics, including seminal figures, key concepts, and emerging trends. Whether you are interested in classical psychoanalysis, object relations theory, or the intersection of neuroscience and psychoanalysis, you will find a wealth of resources within our collection.

One of the hallmarks of our series is its interdisciplinary approach. While rooted in psychoanalytic theory, our volumes draw upon insights from psychology, philosophy, sociology, and other disciplines to offer a holistic understanding of the human mind and its complexities.

Each volume in the series is crafted with the reader in mind, balancing scholarly rigor with engaging prose. Whether you are embarking on your journey into psychoanalysis or seeking to deepen your understanding of specific topics, our series provides a clear and comprehensive roadmap.

Moreover, our series is committed to fostering dialogue and debate within the psychoanalytic community. Each volume invites readers to critically engage with the material, encouraging reflection, discussion, and further exploration.

We invite you to join us on this journey of discovery as we explore the ever-evolving landscape of psychoanalysis.

Aner Govrin

Chapter 1

Introduction

Before We Start

Several books have been published already about online psychotherapy (Derrig-Palumbo & Zeine, 2005; Lemma, 2017; Russell, 2015; Scharff, 2013, 2015, 2017, 2018; Weinberg et al, 2023), so it's only legitimate to ask the question: Why do we need a new one?

The simple answer is that the field of online therapy is developing all the time, especially following the COVID-19 pandemic when everyone had to shift to online sessions. The learning for online therapists from those years (2020–2023) of isolation are invaluable, regarding both research and experience. Most of the above-mentioned books were published beforehand.

The second, no less important, answer is that this book is unique in focusing on using psychoanalytic and psychodynamic approaches online. The books on this topic published following the pandemic did not necessarily focus on psychoanalysis. For example, each of the authors in Weinberg et al.'s book (2023) represented a different school of psychotherapy and described the difficulties each theoretical perspective tackled when moving to online therapy and how their approach influenced the way they overcame these difficulties.

Psychoanalysis as a discipline is usually described and criticized as an old-fashioned approach that has difficulties adjusting itself to the changing world. It seems especially challenging to keep pace with the current rapid technological developments.

DOI: 10.4324/9781003503514-1

Psychoanalysis should review its theory and practice to accommodate these changes. As many authors (e.g., Trub, 2024) pointed out, "the genie is out of the bottle," and we cannot ignore "the elephant in the room." This book is intended to summarize the information about therapy on the internet, describe its implications for psychoanalysis (including how basic analytic dynamics and phenomena emerge in cyberspace), point out the obstacles to doing psychoanalysis online, and help psychodynamic therapists to embrace the online setting.

A Brief History of Online Therapy

Online psychotherapy, a mental health field known as e-therapy or teletherapy, is a form of therapy that takes place over the internet. It allows individuals to participate in therapy sessions from the comfort of their homes, eliminating the need for in-person visits to a therapist's office. The use of online psychotherapy has grown in recent years, especially following the COVID-19 pandemic, as it offers a convenient and accessible alternative to traditional in-person therapy. Nevertheless, there is still a great reluctance among many therapists to use the online modality, especially among psychoanalysts and psychodynamic-oriented therapists, who wonder whether the processes existing in the office, such as transference and resistance, can occur, or are the same, online.

Online therapy has its roots in the late 20th century with the advent of the internet and digital communication technologies. In the 1980s and 1990s, mental health professionals began experimenting with providing therapy services through email and online chat platforms. These early attempts laid the groundwork for what would later become more formalized online therapy platforms. However, its seeds were planted earlier when, for decades, therapists were using the telephone to provide mental health support (Zeavin, 2021).

We can trace the first attempt to create an online session in 1972: During the International Conference on Computers, Stanford and UCLA staff demonstrated a psychotherapy session using linked computers. Although not a real session with a licensed therapist, this event laid the groundwork for the concept of online therapy. Another significant milestone in the development of online therapy was marked in 1986 with the creation of Dear Uncle Ezra, a Cornell University question-and-answer forum. People frequently discussed mental health issues on this platform, although it's unclear whether the responders were licensed therapists. Uncle Ezra was an "anonymous Cornell staffer with a mental health background." In the 1980s and 1990s, mental health professionals began experimenting with providing therapy services through email and online chat platforms. In 1995, therapist John Grohol established Psych Central, which expanded to become a popular mental health publication and forum. At the same time David Sommers pioneered online therapy with continual dialogue and private therapeutic relationships via emails and real-time chats. Clients paid fees for one-on-one therapy.

At the beginning of the 2000s, online therapy gradually gained popularity and became more widespread. With the increasing popularity and accessibility of the internet, dedicated online therapy platforms began to emerge in the early 2000s. These platforms offered a range of services, including text-based therapy, videoconferencing, and forums for support groups. Businesses and therapy practices aimed to treat thousands of clients simultaneously. However, the technology was still unripe for therapists, especially psychodynamically oriented ones, who were hesitant to use videoconferencing since the quality of the video was poor, the picture froze many times, and it disconnected frequently. It was not the last time that technology strongly affected the dynamic processes of the therapy session.

The mid- to late-2000s marked advancements in technology: As technology continued to move forward, online therapy became more sophisticated. Videoconferencing software improved, making it easier for therapists and clients to engage in face-to-face sessions remotely. Additionally, secure messaging platforms and encrypted communication methods enhanced privacy and confidentiality. Throughout the 2010s, online therapy gained greater acceptance among both mental health professionals and the general public. Research studies began to demonstrate the effectiveness of online therapy for various mental health concerns, including depression, anxiety, and post-traumatic stress disorder (PTSD) (Andersson, 2018; Barak et al., 2004; Griffiths et al., 2010; Lange et al, 2003).

There is no doubt that the COVID-19 pandemic accelerated the use, acceptance, and adoption of online therapy, as it offered a convenient and accessible alternative to traditional in-person therapy in times of isolation, and when social distancing measures made in-person sessions more challenging. During the pandemic period (2020–2023), there was a mass transition of therapists to online therapy: According to one survey, an estimate of 98% of therapists used online therapy during the pandemic (Sampaio et al., 2021). In 2023, two-thirds of psychologists surveyed by the American Psychological Association (APA) continued to offer some 35 telepsychological services in their practices, with an additional 21% exclusively offering 36 virtual services (APA, 2023). This vast number of health care professionals working online has created a huge body of experience, knowledge, research, and academic articles (Weinberg et al., 2023). The number of research studies about online therapy jumped exponentially in those three years.

Today, online therapy is often integrated with traditional in-person therapy practices. Many therapists offer a combination of in-person sessions and online sessions to accommodate their clients' needs and preferences. Overall, online therapy has evolved from early experimental efforts to become a mainstream and widely accepted form of mental health treatment, providing accessible and convenient support to individuals around the world. However, it still remains to explore whether psychodynamic psychotherapy, focusing on unconscious processes, can be delivered online, and this book aims to exactly that.

Research About Online Therapy

In recent years, online therapy has garnered increasing attention as a viable and effective alternative to traditional face-to-face therapy. Over the years, studies have explored the effectiveness and implications of online therapy. Below are some key findings.

1. Telepsychology's Efficacy

Several studies have demonstrated the effectiveness of telepsychology. Even before the pandemic erupted, research tested remote care among veterans (Godleski et al., 2012) and a range of age groups and conditions (Hilty et al., 2013), showing that the modality can be effective and increase access to care. Psychologists have also studied a range of populations to determine whether telehealth works, which populations it best serves, and how to deliver it most effectively – with promising results. The U.S. Department of Veterans Affairs, for example, has conducted numerous trials comparing PTSD interventions delivered in person versus by videoconference, finding that the two methods are equally effective in the majority of cases (Turgoose et al., 2018). Systematic reviews have also found that telepsychology delivered by video and phone is effective for depression, anxiety, and adjustment disorder (Varker et al., 2019), as well as for substance use, eating disorders, and other problems in children and adolescents (Slone et al., 2012). Studies also confirmed that remote therapy is as effective as in-person therapy for couples (for example, in low sexual desire couples, Kleinplatz et al., 2024).

2. Meta-Analysis and Randomized Control Trials

The COVID-19 pandemic accelerated research about the effectiveness of online therapy. In a meta-analysis examining pre-post changes within video-delivered psychotherapy (VDP) and comparing the outcomes with in-person psychotherapy (IPP), Fernandez et al. (2021) concluded (p. 1535):

> Substantial and significant improvement occurs from pre- to post-phases of VDP, this in turn differing negligibly from IPP treatment outcome. The VDP improvement … remains strong though attenuated by publication bias. Clinically, therapy is no less efficacious when delivered via videoconferencing than in-person, with efficacy being most pronounced in CBT for affective disorders.

Research using randomized control trials showed that VDP is equally effective as face-to-face psychotherapy in many dimensions, such as client satisfaction (King et al., 2014; Simpson & Reid, 2014) and overall treatment outcome (Kingsley & Henning, 2015; Sucala et al., 2012). The results have been found to be positive for a variety of disorders of *Diagnostic and Statistical Manual of Mental Disorders* (DSM) Axis I, such as depression (Berryhill et al., 2019), anxiety (Backhaus et al., 2012; Chavooshi et al., 2016), and addictions (Backhaus et al., 2012; King et al., 2014), and also for Axis II personality disorders, such as borderline personality disorder (Zimmerman et al., 2021). Giovanetti et al. (2022), who systematically researched databases for research comparing online and offline therapy for depression, claimed that "there is now a sufficiently large corpus of randomized controlled trials to examine the comparative effectiveness of teletherapy and in-person services meta-analytically" (p. 1077). Their conclusion was that video-based teletherapy may be a feasible and effective alternative to in-person services for reducing depressive symptoms. The same result was found by Greenwood et al. (2022) who reviewed randomized controlled trials comparing telehealth versus the face-to-face delivery of psychotherapy for less common mental health conditions and physical health conditions requiring psychotherapy.

In summary, online therapy has proven effective, especially when combined with clinical care.

Advantages and Disadvantages of Online Therapy

Online therapy offers several benefits that make it an appealing option for many individuals.

Advantages

1. Accessibility and Convenience

- *Geographical flexibility*: Online therapy transcends physical boundaries. Clients can access therapy from anywhere. This accessibility eliminates geographical barriers and provides individuals in remote or underserved areas with access to high-quality mental health care. Moreover, individuals with physical disabilities or mobility issues find online therapy particularly beneficial, as it eliminates the need for physical travel and enables them to seek support without hindrance. Thus, it improved access to mental health care.

- *Flexible scheduling*: Sessions can be scheduled to fit the client's availability, making it easier to integrate therapy into a busy lifestyle. With busy schedules and demanding lifestyles becoming the norm, many individuals struggle to find the time for regular therapy sessions. Online therapy addresses this challenge by allowing clients to schedule sessions at their convenience, eliminating the need to rearrange work or personal commitments.

2. *Privacy and Anonymity*

- *Confidentiality*: Conversations are encrypted, and clients can choose anonymous usernames. Through secure messaging platforms and encrypted communication channels, online therapy prioritizes client confidentiality and discretion, creating a safe space for individuals to explore their thoughts and emotions without fear of judgment or exposure. This anonymity encourages open and honest communication between clients and therapists, facilitating more effective therapeutic outcomes and empowering individuals to confront and address their mental health challenges with confidence.
- *Reduced stigma*: Some people find it less intimidating to seek help online, away from the perceived stigma associated with traditional therapy. Online therapy fosters a sense of anonymity and privacy, which is particularly appealing to individuals who may feel stigmatized or apprehensive about seeking therapy.

3. *Comfort and Familiarity*

- *Comfort of home*: Clients can participate in therapy from the comfort of their own homes, reducing anxiety associated with unfamiliar environments.
- *Familiar technology*: Many people, especially younger ones, are accustomed to using digital devices, making online therapy feel natural. However, the technological competency (of both the psychotherapist and the patient) is a crucial factor in providing therapeutic services.

4. Cost Effectiveness

- *Affordability*: Online therapy is often more cost effective than in-person sessions. There are no commuting or parking expenses, and some platforms offer lower fees. Traditional therapy can be prohibitively expensive, with session fees, transportation costs, and time commitments adding up over the periods of therapy. In contrast, online therapy often offers more affordable rates and flexible payment options, making mental health care accessible to a broader spectrum of individuals. This affordability democratizes mental health care, ensuring that individuals from all socioeconomic backgrounds can access the support they need to thrive.

5. Increased Options

- *Variety of therapists*: Clients can choose from a diverse pool of therapists, including those with specialized expertise.
- *Multiple modalities*: Online therapy encompasses various formats, such as chat, video calls, and phone calls.

6. Consistent Support

- *Asynchronous communication*: Messaging-based therapy allows clients to express themselves at their own pace, fostering consistent communication.
- *Crisis support*: Some platforms offer 24/7 crisis chat services.

7. Reduced Wait Times

- *Immediate access*: Clients can often start therapy sooner than with traditional in-person services, which may have long waiting lists.

In conclusion, the advantages of online therapy are manifold, ranging from enhanced accessibility and convenience to cost effectiveness and privacy. By leveraging digital technologies and innovative platforms, online therapy has transcended traditional barriers to mental health care, empowering individuals to prioritize their well-being on their own terms. As society continues to embrace the digital age, online therapy represents a paradigm shift in mental health treatment, offering a transformative approach that is inclusive, accessible, and empowering for all.

We should remember that while online therapy has numerous advantages, its quality depends on choosing a reputable platform and a qualified therapist to ensure a positive experience.

Disadvantages

While online therapy has its advantages, it also comes with some disadvantages that individuals should consider.

1. Lack of Nonverbal Cues

- *Nonverbal cues*: One of the primary drawbacks of online therapy is the potential loss of nonverbal cues and interpersonal dynamics inherent in face-to-face interactions (Weinberg, 2020a). Unlike traditional therapy, where therapists can observe clients' body language, facial expressions, and subtle cues, online therapy often relies solely on verbal communication through videoconferencing or text-based platforms. This limitation can impede the therapeutic process, as therapists may miss important contextual information and struggle to fully understand clients' emotions and experiences. The nonverbal cues, like body language, facial expressions, and tone of voice cues are essential for understanding emotions and building rapport.

2. Technical Challenges

- *Technical and connectivity issues*: Poor internet connections can disrupt sessions, affecting the quality of communication. They can also cause video freezes, audio delays, or dropped calls, which can be frustrating for both clients and therapists. From a psychodynamic perspective, some clients, who are sensitive to abandonment issues, can react strongly to dropping the connection. Technological glitches and connectivity issues further hinder effective communication and rapport-building between clients and therapists.

- *Technological literacy and cultural issues*: The effectiveness of online therapy may be influenced by factors such as technological literacy, access to reliable internet connectivity, and cultural considerations. Individuals who are not familiar with digital technologies (such as older people) or who lack access to high-speed internet may struggle to engage effectively in online therapy sessions, limiting their ability to benefit from treatment. Moreover, cultural differences in communication styles and therapeutic norms may pose challenges in establishing rapport and understanding between clients and therapists from diverse backgrounds.

3. Security and Privacy Concerns

- *Data privacy*: Although platforms prioritize confidentiality, data breaches or privacy violations are possible. Despite advancements in encryption and secure communication technologies, online therapy platforms may still be vulnerable to data breaches, hacking, and unauthorized access. Clients may feel hesitant to disclose sensitive personal information or discuss sensitive topics online, fearing that their privacy may be compromised.
- *Client's environment*: Clients must ensure a private and secure environment for therapy sessions. The lack of physical confidentiality in online therapy settings raises concerns about the confidentiality of therapy sessions, as clients may be overheard or interrupted by household members or co-workers.

4. Limited Crisis Intervention

- *Delayed responses*: Asynchronous communication (e.g., messaging) may not provide immediate crisis support.
- *Emergency situations*: In urgent cases, online therapy may not be as effective as face-to-face interventions. While online therapy can effectively address common concerns such as

depression, anxiety, and stress, it may lack the comprehensive support and intervention necessary for managing severe psychiatric disorders or acute crises. In psychodynamic terms, in these situations, the severely distressed client needs a physical holding environment that is lacking in cyberspace. In such cases, face-to-face therapy or inpatient treatment may be more appropriate, as they offer immediate access to intensive care and crisis intervention services that online therapy cannot provide.

5. Not Suitable for All Conditions

- *Severe mental health issues*: Online therapy may not be appropriate for severe or complex mental health conditions, such as psychosis or acute suicidal thoughts, that require intensive or specialized treatment (or at least needs special expertise/training on how to provide the appropriate service online for such cases).
- *Complex cases*: Some cases require in-person assessments and interventions.

6. Depersonalization

- *Digital disconnect*: Clients might feel less connected due to the absence of physical presence. This phenomenon can exacerbate when clients hold an avoidant-dismissive attachment style or tend to dissociate under stressful conditions due to previous traumas.
- *Less personal interaction*: Online interactions can feel transactional rather than deeply personal. For psychodynamic therapists, who focus on relationship development in the sessions and the transference-countertransference matrix, this can cause a serious limitation.

7. Ethical Challenges

- *Boundary management*: Therapists must set clear boundaries regarding response times and availability.

- *Dual relationships*: Online platforms can blur professional and personal boundaries. The fact that the therapist might also connect from home poses a challenge for the privacy of the therapist.

8. Lack of Regulation

- *Varied standards*: Online therapy lacks consistent regulations across platforms and countries.
- *Quality control*: Not all therapists offering online services are equally qualified or effective.

9. Screen Fatigue

- *Zoom fatigue*: Constant screen time can lead to mental fatigue and burnout.

10. Loss of In-Person Benefits

- *Lack of human connection*: Some clients (and many therapists, certainly psychoanalysts) value the warmth and presence of face-to-face interactions.
- *Environmental change*: Leaving home for therapy sessions provides a change of environment.

The shift to online psychotherapy introduces heightened risks of regulatory and ethical breaches. Practicing across jurisdictions can easily lead clinicians to provide services outside the scope of their licensure or geographic authority, particularly when national or regional regulations differ or are poorly understood. Moreover, therapists may inadvertently operate beyond their area of clinical competence, especially when transitioning to digital modalities without adequate training. For patients, it becomes more difficult to verify the therapist's credentials, licensure status, or professional reputation, especially when selecting providers from online directories or commercial platforms. Compounding these concerns, some digital therapy platforms act as intermediaries in the therapeutic contract, holding control over access and communication.

This has, in some cases, resulted in abrupt service disruptions when platforms change policies, deactivate providers, or cease operations, all without sufficient notice or recourse for patients or therapists.

In conclusion, while online therapy offers valuable benefits in terms of accessibility, convenience, and affordability, it is essential to recognize and address its limitations. From the loss of nonverbal cues and interpersonal dynamics to concerns about privacy and security, online therapy presents unique challenges that require careful consideration and mitigation strategies. By acknowledging these limitations and adopting evidence-based practices, mental health professionals can maximize the efficacy and impact of online therapy while ensuring that clients receive the support and care they need to thrive. The bottom line is that the suitability of online therapy depends on individual preferences, needs, and severity of their mental health concerns.

Overcoming the Challenges of Online Therapy

The challenges and obstacles in online therapy call for creative solutions to overcome them. Some of the difficulties in finding such solutions stem from the expectations that online therapy should be the same as in-person therapy. If we take this idea to the extreme, therapists who use the psychoanalytic couch in their office should insist that the patient lie on the couch in front of the computer screen, which seems quite strange. In the introduction to their edited book *Advances in Online Therapy: Emergence of a New Paradigm* (2023), Weinberg et al. recommend applying flexibility and creativity when moving from the couch to the screen. They write (p. 3):

> If we want to adjust ourselves to the new conditions of online therapy, we must be flexible, especially regarding the setting and boundaries of the sessions. This flexibility negates the long tradition of psychodynamic psychotherapy, which assumes that the therapist should establish rigid boundaries in order to guarantee a better holding environment.

One of the main changes between the online setting and offline one is that at least half of the online setting is determined by the patients (they choose a quiet room with privacy), so therapists should abandon the notion that they are the only ones controlling the setting and acknowledge that they share responsibility with the patients for creating a safe environment. This means that the therapist should prepare the patient for the online setting and instruct them how to take care of the surroundings in their room to create a holding environment. For example, reminding them that they should guarantee the use of a quiet, private room. However, from a psychodynamic point of view, this means that the therapist recruits the patient's ego functions and strength, and that it might prevent some deeper regression, which is needed to get in touch with unconscious material. Another difficulty that this appeal for flexibility causes is the question "How flexible should we become?". It is easier to work in a clear frame of reference that recommends strict boundaries, and it might be confusing to adjust to new and more flexible boundaries online. For example, should the therapist connect from their office every time? If they connect from their home, what to do with the inadvertent self-disclosure? Should the therapist create a virtual fake background or blur the background as some online applications allow them to do?

We will discuss further the meaning and importance of the setting in the psychoanalytic frame of reference in the next chapter, Chapter 2, where we describe the features of psychoanalytic/psychodynamic treatment. In the meantime, we should acknowledge that the therapist's role is to ensure uninterrupted sessions and a comfortable setting with patients to maximize the impact of the sessions. Establishing the therapeutic frame in online therapy requires deliberate attention to recreate the structure of in-person therapeutic interactions within a virtual environment. It is crucial to foster an open dialogue with patients about the online process, including guidelines for communication and boundaries.

Weinberg (2020a, 2021) argues that online therapy presents specific challenges, which training can help therapists consider and overcome. Some of these obstacles can be overcome and compensated for by flexibility (e.g., the changed setting), whereas others should be acknowledged as losses and only partially overcome by creativity (e.g., the absence of body-to-body interactions). Thus, creativity is another important factor in overcoming the obstacles of online therapy. For example, Geller (2023) suggested creative ways to cultivate a therapeutic presence online (e.g., experiment with different distances from the screen with patients, to ascertain what feels comfortable and present for them), and Weinberg (2020a) recommended increasing self-disclosure and transparency of therapists to create their online presence.

The Scope of This Book

This book focuses on the application of psychoanalytic and psychodynamic therapy to the online setting. First, it summarizes the current state of affairs in the field of online psychotherapy and covers up-to-date research about the impact of online therapy compared to in-person therapy, especially looking at the topic of the therapeutic alliance, which is the main factor positively correlated with a successful therapeutic outcome. The book describes the main characteristics of the psychodynamic approach (transference, countertransference, resistance, dream interpretation, etc.) and explores the ways in which those psychodynamic processes exist online. It not only focuses on the fact that technology has become part of the transference-countertransference matrix but also highlights the practices for therapists conducting online therapy sessions, such as managing boundaries and maintaining confidentiality and privacy.

In addition, this book relates to different formats of online therapy: Individual, couple, and group therapy. The need for training in this specific field is discussed, and the author suggests an outline of appropriate training for online therapy. Finally, the book concludes with an attempt to predict the future of online psychodynamic psychotherapy.

A few books have already been written on this specific subject beyond the general literature on online psychotherapy: Jill Scharff (2013, 2015, 2017, 2018) edited a series of four books entitled Psychotherapy Online. Each volume offers a discussion on the significance of remote treatment and how it affects the therapeutic relationship. Other relevant books are *Distance Psychoanalysis* (Carlino, 2011), *Screen Relations* (Russell, 2015), and *The Digital Age on the Couch* (Lemma, 2017), and there was also a special issue of the journal, Psychoanalytic Perspectives (2017). However, all these books were written and published before the COVID-19 pandemic. The pandemic had a huge impact on online therapy, including online psychodynamic therapy, since almost all psychoanalysts and psychodynamically oriented therapists moved online, and the experience and research accumulated in the three years of the pandemic are invaluable. This book tries to fill this gap and share the new knowledge following the pandemic.

I need to clarify that, in this book, I propose an evolution, not a deviation: The online modality is not intended to replace in-person meetings. Whenever it is possible, I recommend integrating online sessions with periodic in-person meetings. This hybrid structure carefully preserves the embodied experience that is so central to the psychoanalytic tradition while expanding access and ensuring that this discipline remains responsive to the realities of an interconnected, post-pandemic world.

Chapter 2

What Is Psychoanalytic-Oriented Psychotherapy

Psychoanalytic vs. Psychodynamic Psychotherapy

Psychoanalytic therapy and psychodynamic therapy are both rooted in the principles established by Sigmund Freud and focus on exploring the unconscious mind, childhood experiences, and the therapeutic relationship. Both these approaches focus on the unconscious and seek to explore unconscious thoughts and feelings that influence behavior. However, there are some differences between the two, especially concerning therapeutic techniques. Below are the main features that distinguish these two approaches.

Psychoanalytic Therapy

1 *Depth of exploration*: Psychoanalysis involves a deep and comprehensive exploration of the unconscious mind.
2 *Long-term*: It is typically a long-term process, often lasting several years with multiple sessions per week.
3 *Techniques*: It utilizes techniques such as free association, dream analysis, and interpretation of resistance and transference.
4 *Therapist's role*: The therapist often maintains a neutral stance, allowing the patient to project thoughts and feelings onto them.
5 *Intensive process*: It involves frequent sessions (three to five times per week), requiring a significant time commitment from the patient.
6 *Use of the couch*: The patient usually lies on the couch with the analyst sitting behind.

DOI: 10.4324/9781003503514-2

Psychodynamic Therapy (Gabbard, 2010)

1 *Shorter duration*: Typically, psychodynamic therapy is shorter-term compared to traditional psychoanalysis, often lasting a few months.
2 *Therapeutic relationship*: The relationship between the therapist and the patient is crucial, with a focus on transference and countertransference.
3 *Past experiences*: While it examines past experiences, it is more focused in the present, looking at how past events shape current behavior.
4 *Less intensive*: Sessions are generally once a week, making them less intensive than psychoanalytic therapy.
5 *Use of the couch*: This is usually unnecessary in psychodynamic therapy.
6 *Goal-oriented*: Aims to improve self-awareness and understand the influence of the past on present behavior.

Throughout this book, I use psychoanalytic and psychodynamic psychotherapy interchangeably, despite the differences mentioned above, since the similarities outweigh the differences.

Different Psychoanalytic Schools

To explore whether psychoanalytic/psychodynamic psychotherapy can be applied online, we must first define the characteristics of this approach to therapy. This seemingly easy task becomes complicated because more than one psychodynamic approach has been developed since Freud established psychoanalysis at the beginning of the 20th century. The American Psychoanalytic Association's (APsA's) website (APsA, n.d.) claims that the major therapeutic perspective transplanted to the United States was ego psychology, centrally based on Sigmund Freud's *The Ego and the Id* (1923), followed by Anna Freud's *Ego and the Mechanisms of Defense* (1936) and Heinz Hartmann's *Ego Psychology and the Problem of Adaptation* (1958). Meanwhile, in Europe, the major theoretical approach that has been developed was Object Relations, established by Melanie Klein (1923, 1935) and developed further by Fairbairn (1953). The "Independent" group of British analysts, such as Winnicott (1965) moved away from the Kleinian group. This picture became more confused in 1971, when Heinz Kohut's book, *The Psychology of the Self*, inaugurated a new theoretical perspective in American psychoanalysis: Self-psychology. This new approach paved the way to the relational approaches (Greenberg and Mitchell, 1983) that emerged in the United States and other parts of the world toward the end of the 20th century.

It is not easy to describe the main features that distinguish each of the psychoanalytic approaches from one another, and the scope of this book does not allow a detailed description. Instead, below is a very brief summary of each of the main psychoanalytic and psychodynamic approaches and their main features.

- *Classical psychoanalysis*:
  - Is based on drive theory; drives (such as sex and aggression) are behind every behavior.
  - Focuses on id and oedipal issues.
- *Ego psychology*:
  - Reminds us that there is a conflict-free ego sphere.
  - Focuses on coping and adaptation.
- *Object relations*:
  - Shift from drive to object relations.
  - Shift from oedipal to pre-oedipal issues.
  - Explores how people develop their psyche in relation to important objects in their environment, especially during infancy.
- *Self-psychology*:
  - Has emphasis on empathy and (real) empathic failure of the therapist.
  - A stable sense of self develops through empathic relationships with other people, or "self-objects." Self-objects meet the developing self's needs for mirroring, idealization, and twinship.

- *Relational/intersubjective approaches*:
  - Consider that the therapist has an unconscious mind; thus, we should talk about the transference-countertransference matrix, and not talk about these separately.
  - Emphasise the co-construction of behavior by both therapist and patient.

So the question to be considered is what the common features of all these theories are. It looks as if every psychodynamic theory emphasizes unconscious processes and unresolved past conflicts as influencing behavior. There are also common features in the therapeutic technique. The key common elements are:

1 *Tripartite personality* (Kernberg, 2016):
  - Personality consists of three structures – id, ego, and superego.
  - These structures interact and shape behavior.

2 *Psychosexual stages*:
  - Freud proposed stages (oral, anal, phallic, latent, genital) where conflicts arise.
  - Unresolved conflicts impact personality development.

3 *Unconscious mind* (Freud, 1915):
  - Behavior is influenced by hidden desires, memories, and emotions. The unconscious mind is shaping thoughts, feelings, and behaviors.
  - The therapist studies the unconscious mind to identify and release repressed thoughts, feelings, and desires that may be negatively impacting a person's life.
  - Dreams and slips of the tongue reveal unconscious content. The therapist uses dreams, fantasies, and play to suggest hidden aspects of a patient's psyche.
  - Free association (saying the first thing that comes to mind without censoring it) can help identify hidden thoughts and experiences.

4 *Defense mechanisms*:

- The ego uses defense mechanisms (e.g., repression, projection) to cope with anxiety.
- These protect against threatening thoughts.

5 *Exploration of childhood experiences*:

- Early childhood experiences significantly influence adult personality and behavior.
- Therapy aims to uncover and work through unresolved issues from the past.

6 *Therapeutic relationship*:

- The quality of the therapeutic relationship is crucial. A person's relationships, including with their psychoanalyst, may include elements from their earliest relationships.
- The therapist serves as a blank screen onto which the client can project feelings, providing a safe space to explore emotions and thoughts (the relational approaches disagree with this notion).

7 *Insight and self-understanding*:

- The goal in therapy is to increase self-awareness and insight into unconscious patterns of thinking and behaving, leading to personal growth and change.
- Interpretation and analysis: Therapists interpret clients' thoughts, feelings, and behaviors to uncover underlying meanings and unconscious processes.

8 *Long-term treatment*:

- Typically, long-term treatments delve deep into the client's psyche to address underlying issues comprehensively.

Other important concepts, such as the holding environment, the setting, and the therapeutic alliance, are relevant for all psychodynamic approaches. Let us discuss each of them and their relevance to online treatment.

The Holding Environment

From the above description, it seems that the difficulty in shifting from the couch to the screen does not lie in the theoretical field. Conceptualizing the three parts of the personality, perceiving human development according to psychosexual stages, and acknowledging the existence of unconscious processes, do not change when we work online. The main difficulty seems to be with the technique, especially the setting, which changes dramatically when we move online. The question is whether we can create the same holding environment that encourages the exploration of these unconscious processes, enables the development of therapeutic alliance, transference, and countertransference, and facilitates self-awareness and insight.

Winnicott (1965) described the holding environment as the total environmental provision for an infant. He extended the concept from mother-infant relationships to the therapeutic setting. The key aspects of the therapeutic holding environment are containment, empathy, patience, authenticity, and abstinence. To explore the question of whether we can create this holding environment online, let us look at the 12 requirements that Winnicott (1955) listed for a safe holding environment that enables psychoanalytic treatment.

1. The analyst puts themself at the service of the patient at a certain time convenient to both parties. This can be arranged online or offline.
2. The analyst would be reliable by being there at every meeting, alive and breathing. Surely the online setting does not hinder it.
3. For the length of the scheduled meeting, the analyst should become preoccupied with the patient and stay awake. It might be more challenging online since it is easier to become distractible, but with appropriate training and discipline, it can be achieved.
4. Love and hate should be expressed honestly by the analyst: Love by a genuine positive interest in the patient and hate as a firm maintenance of reality and separateness – the therapist's refusal to be omnipotent, infinitely available, or self-sacrificing. Both love and hate as described by Winnicott, can be expressed online.

5 The analyst must genuinely connect with the patient's emotional experience, try to understand it, and communicate this understanding in words. Resistance means that the patient suffers, but it can be alleviated by interpretation. Since the analyst continues to communicate verbally online, the analyst can still do the above on the internet. Connecting with the patient's emotional experience might be more challenging online but can be learned.
6 The analyst's method is the objective interpretation, which can be done online
7 The work is to be done in a quiet room (but not completely quiet) that is properly lit and comfortably warm. The patient should lie on a couch. Here we have the biggest challenge regarding the setting that certainly needs adjustment, just as lying on the couch is not a requirement anymore in psychodynamic psychotherapy. In Chapter 1, I mentioned that we can teach the patient how to take care of having the use of a quiet, private, and comfortable room. Since this is one of the main difficulties in psychoanalysis online, I will refer to it in a separate paragraph below.
8 Neutral and abstaining attitude: Avoiding imposing the analyst's own views or interpretations. The analyst should keep moral judgment out of the meeting and should not take sides. They should accept the patient unconditionally. This requirement is not affected by the online conditions.
9 The analyst is reliable: They should be free from temper tantrums, be patient, and be punctual. This allows the patient to unfold their thoughts and feelings at their own pace. Reliability does not depend on the media.
10 There should be a clear distinction between fact and fantasy, which allows freedom for the patient to fantasize anything they wish, from aggressive to sexual desires. Fantasy is an internal process, and the analyst can create the safety to express it online as well.
11 There should be no retaliation from the analyst. This allows the patient to express aggression and try to destroy the analyst (who survives). Online, it is easier for the analyst to keep this attitude since the screen provides more protection.
12 The analyst survives. As said, it is less challenging for the analyst to survive online.

The Setting

When referring to the setting in psychodynamic work, it means all the characteristics of the framework and the laws that are intended to ensure *a priori* the environmental conditions necessary for the existence and effective conduct of the act of treatment. The setting is intended to protect the interests of both the patient and the therapist in a way that will advance the work of the act of therapy and guarantee and secure it as much as possible against disturbances, whether conscious or unconscious. It is a combination of concrete and subjective elements in the psychotherapy framework that are set up to provide continuity, consistency, and containment. A stable and safe environment helps patients feel free to explore and express their minds.

The setting is considered the essential background that provides containment and allows transference and unconscious processes to emerge. Freud writes in detail about the rules for the analytic setting, including temporal aspects (such as time, length, and frequency of meetings), space aspects (place and conditions in the room), financial aspects, and the analyst's position (abstinence, neutrality and anonymity). Langs (1998) dedicated an entire book to the setting and frame of the analytic situation. Bleger (1967/2018) commented that the analytic situation is defined as a process, but, as with any process, it needs a stable variable, which is the setting. He adds that we notice the setting only when it is disrupted. Modell (1989) sees the therapeutic setting as creating a warm, womb-like, safe, and containing space, protecting the patient from the difficult reality outside the room.

To examine whether the stable setting can be kept online and continue to provide continuity, consistency and containment, we follow Triest's two principles conceptualizations of the setting (2011). The first (in the order of development of psychoanalysis as well) covers the formal aspects ("the law of the father"). It includes meeting time, duration, frequency, payment, and method of payment. The way to ensure this aspect of the setting from the therapist's side is to keep the neutrality, anonymity, and abstinence of the therapist. Most of these rigid elements of the setting do not change in online therapy (or can easily be obtained), and sometimes they are even helped by shifting online (e.g., abstinence). As said, to ensure the boundaries of the setting at the patient's end, the therapist should simply instruct the patient to guarantee the use of a quiet room and keep the privacy of the meetings. Weiner and Bornstein (2009) deal with the construction of the therapeutic contract in the initial phase of the treatment. In order for the therapeutic contract to be successful, they suggest that it must be understandable, explicit, and agreed upon by both parties. This can be done online usually in the first online meeting or the intake.

As for the second conceptualization of the setting, with Winnicott's ideas, the concept of the framework became more focused on the mother figure (the "mother" figure has expanded to the maternal or the major caregiver role). The holding environment was conceived as a womb, warm, safe, containing, and protected from the outside world. Since holding is based on the actual hands of the mother, hugging and encompassing the baby, this aspect is usually the one that psychoanalytic-oriented therapists are concerned about while moving online. Usually, they express this concern by doubting whether they can create the appropriate presence in online meetings (Lemma 2017; Russell 2015). The presence of the therapist involves their immersion, passion, attention, emotional involvement, reverie, and a readiness to be drawn into enactments (Grossmark, 2007). Lemma (2017) writes that presence is the perception of successfully transforming an intention into action, and actions are not restricted to ones that we discharge physically. In their book about therapeutic presence, Geller and Greenberg (2012) describe therapeutic presence as the state of having one's whole self in the encounter with a client or a group by being completely in the moment on a multiplicity of levels – physically, emotionally, cognitively, and spiritually. As said before, there are ways to cultivate therapeutic presence online (Geller, 2023; Weinberg, 2020a), although it requires special training.

I would like to argue that when we discuss whether a good-enough holding environment, an appropriate setting, or adequate presence can exist online, we miss a central point: The important factor that determines the quality of psychodynamic psychotherapy is whether we listen to the unconscious communication as it responds to the setting and the changes that apply to it. The psychodynamic therapist should be attuned to the reactions of the patient to the changes in the setting, both the conscious and unconscious ones, and discuss these emotional and psychological responses (and their implications) with the patient. This is the essence of the therapeutic psychoanalytic process, and it should be maintained in online treatment.

Time Boundaries

Time boundaries are an essential element of the setting. However, "electronic" time can be different from "clock" time outside the computer. In online therapy, there are different dynamics around the beginning of sessions than with in-person meetings. If the therapist activates the "waiting room" option on the meeting application, the experience of the patient waiting to be called in is not the same as in the waiting room at the office. The patient feels more like being "kept out" and not allowed into the session. In case they come early and wait in the virtual waiting room, the option of seeing the therapist's previous patient disappears, which affects the dynamics of competition and envy. Since the patient connects from home, arriving, whether early, on time, or late, has different meanings in the online world. Kegerreis (2022) considers how difficult it is to take up these dynamics adequately when faced with the real uncertainties of internet connections, or any other technical issues, such as computer restarting, apps reloading, updating, etc. The way sessions end is also very different. When the therapist ends the session, it feels as if it is cut with an axe since it's an abrupt disconnection. The experience of time within sessions is altered, and sessions are no longer bracketed with the journey to and from the consulting room.

Therapeutic Alliance

The therapeutic alliance is a crucial component in psychodynamic therapy. It refers to the collaborative and trusting relationship between the therapist and the client, which is essential for effective treatment. In psychodynamic therapy, the therapeutic alliance facilitates the exploration of unconscious processes, internal conflicts, and relational patterns that influence the client's psychological well-being.

Key elements of the therapeutic alliance include:

1. *Bonding*: The emotional connection between therapist and client, characterized by trust, empathy, and respect.
2. *Agreement on goals*: Shared understanding and consensus on the goals of therapy and the focus of the work.
3. *Agreement on tasks*: Mutual agreement on the methods and interventions used during therapy to achieve the established goals.

Research has consistently shown that a strong therapeutic alliance is associated with better treatment outcomes across various therapeutic modalities, including psychodynamic therapy. For example, a meta-analysis by Horvath and Symonds (1991) found a moderate to large effect size for the relationship between the quality of the therapeutic alliance and therapy outcomes. Similarly, studies by Safran and Muran (2000) highlight the importance of the alliance in facilitating the resolution of intrapsychic conflicts and fostering self-awareness, which are central to psychodynamic work.

In psychodynamic therapy specifically, the therapeutic alliance enables the client to feel safe enough to explore deep-seated and often distressing material, such as early attachment patterns and unresolved conflicts. This safe space helps clients to rework these issues within the therapeutic relationship, which can lead to meaningful changes in their psychological functioning and interpersonal relationships.

Does therapeutic alliance exist in online therapy? Research results mentioned in the previous chapter show no significant difference between online and offline therapy, which can be explained by the existence of the therapeutic alliance online as an intermediate variable. The last two factors of the alliance (agreeing on the goals and tasks) can easily be achieved online by discussing the goals and tasks before beginning therapy (e.g. in the online first meeting). The concern is that technology impacts the first factor of bonding. However, studies examining clients' perceptions of the therapeutic alliance using telehealth found that a workable therapeutic alliance is possible to achieve (Rasmussen et al., 2022). In some studies, the therapeutic alliance was reported to be equally as strong as in-person settings (Flückiger et al., 2020; Simpson & Reid, 2014).

By embracing effective communication strategies and navigating environmental factors with proficiency and foresight, psychodynamic therapists can create inclusive and accessible therapeutic environments. According to Shoullis et al. (2023), what helps the therapeutic alliance navigate the change of frame are the innovation of new ways of working collaboratively, the prior establishment of a bond in person, and the consistent maintenance of other aspects of the frame.

Shedler's Seven Factors Applied Online

As a final step in exploring the possibility of online psychodynamic therapy, let us examine Shedler's seven factors of psychodynamic psychotherapy. Shedler (2010) suggested that all psychodynamic approaches include seven common elements. We will check whether each of them can be applied online.

1. *Focus on affect and expression of emotion*

> Psychodynamic therapy encourages exploration and discussion of the full range of a patient's emotions. The therapist helps the patient describe and put words to feelings, including contradictory feelings, feelings that are troubling or threatening, and feelings that the patient may not initially be able to recognize or acknowledge
>
> (Shedler, 2010, p. 99)

The online psychodynamic therapist can certainly encourage the exploration of the full range of emotions.

2. *Exploration of attempts to avoid distressing thoughts and feelings*

> Defenses and resistance can be open, such as missing sessions or arriving late, or more subtle. Psychodynamic therapists

actively focus on and explore avoidance. Online, there are additional ways to avoid thoughts and feelings and to express resistance (e.g., turning off the video), however a skilled therapist can notice these overt and subtle ways and explore them.

3. *Identification of recurring themes and patterns*

   Identifying and exploring recurring themes in patients' thoughts, feelings, self-concept, and relationships can reveal self-defeating patterns and behaviors. Patients may be unaware of the patterns until the therapist helps them. Again, online communication does not pose any limitations to this exploration.

4. *Exploration of past experiences*

   Past experiences, especially early ones of attachment figures, affect our relation to the present. Exploring early experiences and the relation between past and present helps patients free themselves from the bonds of the past. This can occur online and offline.

5. *Focus on interpersonal relations*

   Psychodynamic therapists emphasize patients' relationships, their object relations, and attachment. Psychological difficulties arise when problematic interpersonal patterns interfere with the fulfillment of patients' emotional needs. Interpersonal relationships can be explored online and offline.

6. *Focus on the therapy relationship*

   In the psychodynamic frame of reference, we focus on the relationship between therapist and patient, and how it is affected by past relationship with caregivers, meaning, on transference. This examination of the repetition of interpersonal themes in the therapy relationship and the therapist's reaction to them (transference and countertransference) provides an opportunity to explore the patient's relationship in the world and change them in the room. As we will see in Chapter 4, transference can also develop online (Eichenberger & Boswell, 2024) but, when examining it, we should include the impact of the remote relationship on it.

7. *Exploration of fantasy life*

In psychodynamic therapy, the therapist uses free association, encouraging patients to speak freely about whatever is on their minds. This material is a rich source of information about how the person views self and others, interprets and makes sense of experience, avoids aspects of experience, or interferes with a potential capacity to find greater enjoyment and meaning in life. This exploration of fantasy life can be achieved online as well, by creating the safe container.

Kranzberg (1986) suggested that technological developments are not intrinsically good or bad, but neither are they neutral. I suggest following his ideas.

Chapter 3

The Body in Psychoanalysis

Introduction

Psychoanalysis holds a complicated position regarding the importance of the body in the human psyche and its central position in psychodynamic psychotherapy. Since this book is about online psychodynamic psychotherapy, where one of the clearly missing elements is the body (or, actually, the body-to-body interaction), it is imperative that we examine how psychoanalysts relate to the body in therapy, both theoretically and practically/technically.

Technically Speaking

Freud's early technique of touching the patient's forehead, known as the "pressure technique," was part of his initial method in the late 1880s and early 1890s, before the full development of psychoanalysis. He sought a way to access repressed memories quickly. He would place his hand on the patient's forehead and ask them to recall a specific memory or association, while applying gentle pressure. Freud (1895) believed this act would help the patient overcome resistance and bring unconscious material to consciousness. It was both a symbolic and a physical gesture intended to convey authority and focus attention. This method was a precursor to the free association technique, which Freud later developed as he abandoned more directive approaches in favor of letting the patient's psyche unfold naturally. The forehead-touching technique gradually fell out of use as Freud realized that

DOI: 10.4324/9781003503514-3

allowing patients to speak freely without interruption led to deeper insights and more enduring therapeutic results.

The free association technique is related to the use of the couch in psychoanalysis. Lying on the couch was a tool to foster free association and reduce external distractions. Freud (1913) asked patients to lie on a couch, with him seated behind them, out of sight (notice the lack of eye-to-eye contact in Freud's original technique, which is one of the features criticized as missing online by those who object to online psychoanalysis).

This physical arrangement served several key purposes:

1 *Encouraging free association*: By not facing the analyst, patients felt freer to speak without censorship or concern for the analyst's facial expressions or judgments.
2 *Reducing transference distortions*: It allowed unconscious feelings and projections (transference) to emerge more clearly, unfiltered by the analyst's visible presence.
3 *Minimizing visual stimuli*: Lying down in a relaxed position without making eye contact helped patients access deeper layers of their unconscious.
4 *Symbolizing regression*: The posture invoked a more childlike, regressed state, making it easier to access early developmental material.

So, on the one hand, from the technical perspective, Freud shifted to less and less touch and body/face-to-face presence in his practice, recommending the rule of abstinence as a foundational principle in classical Freudian psychoanalysis. This rule refers to the analyst's stance of withholding gratification from the patient during treatment, particularly emotional, physical, or behavioral comforts that could ease psychological tension prematurely. The analyst does not act on the patient's desires for love or parental comfort – avoiding hugs and refusing to hold the patient's hand or to gratify any physical contact. This rule, together with avoiding eye contact while lying on the couch, suits the online modality well, as there is no body gratification and it is difficult to establish eye-to-eye contact.

Theoretically Speaking

At the same time, from a theoretical point of view, Freud emphasized the role of the body in the development of the ego. He proposed that the ego – the sense of "I" or self – originates from the body, particularly from how the infant experiences bodily sensations and bodily boundaries. This concept (the first ego is a body ego) is a foundational psychoanalytic insight into how the self (ego) emerges through early bodily experiences. The body ego develops as the infant becomes aware of the physical self through sensations such as hunger, touch, pleasure, and pain. These bodily experiences provide the raw material for the formation of the ego. He writes: The ego is first and foremost a bodily ego; it is not merely a surface entity but is itself the projection of a surface (Freud, 1923, p. 26). This means the ego begins as a mental representation of the body, especially the body's surface, its skin and sensory boundaries, through which the infant starts to distinguish between self and non-self, inside and outside.

Later theorists such as Didier Anzieu (1985) and Donald Winnicott (1960) expanded on this idea, exploring how the body ego contributes to identity formation, self-containment, and the experience of the psyche as "held" in a body. In his influential book *Le Moi-Peau* (*The Skin Ego*, 1985), Anzieu elaborates on Freud's body ego by proposing that the skin functions as a psychic envelope – a kind of metaphorical container for the ego. His central thesis is that the skin is experienced by the infant as the boundary of the self, and this sensory and tactile experience is internalized to become a psychological structure: The "skin ego." As mentioned above, when we discussed the holding environment, while Winnicott did not use the term "skin ego," his concept of the holding environment aligns with Anzieu's ideas. He emphasized that the caregiver's physical and emotional "holding" of the infant helps build the ego's sense of safety and integrity.

The Still Face – Criticism About the Missing Body in Psychoanalysis and Online Therapy

How do these ideas align with the absence of bodily interactions in the psychoanalytic technique? Many contemporary psychoanalysts (e.g., relational and intersubjective theorists) have reconsidered its rigidity: Heinz Kohut and self-psychologists warned that excessive abstinence can retraumatize narcissistically wounded patients. Relational analysts (e.g., Mitchell, 1988) argue for a more mutual, responsive engagement, where some emotional attunement or limited gratification can actually deepen the analytic process.

From a research point of view, The Still Face experiment by Ed Tronick et al. (1978) has had profound implications for developmental psychology and, increasingly, for psychoanalysis, especially in light of challenges posed by online therapy and the absence of physical presence, gaze, and touch. In the experiment, a mother interacts with her infant as usual: Cooing, smiling, responding. Then, she suddenly adopts a still, neutral, unresponsive face. The baby quickly becomes distressed, making increasingly desperate attempts to re-engage her through smiles, gestures, vocalizations, before eventually withdrawing or showing signs of dysregulation.

This demonstrated that infants expect attuned, contingent responses from caregivers, and that even brief relational disruptions provoke anxiety and loss of coherence in the self. Tronick's findings underscore how bodily presence, facial mirroring, and mutual gaze are foundational to human regulation and emotional development (Tronick et al., 1978). In traditional psychoanalysis, these bodily cues are minimized (e.g., the patient on the couch, the analyst out of view), but the therapist's embodied presence is still subtly registered through breathing, pauses, tone, and posture. Online psychoanalysis reduces or eliminates these sensory cues, raising concerns about missing attunement, micro-disruptions (echoes of the "still face") and mis-attunement being misinterpreted as withdrawal or disinterest. Tronick et al. (1978) also showed that affect regulation is co-created: The baby relies on the caregiver to modulate emotional states. Similarly, in psychoanalysis, the analyst functions as a regulatory other, a "second skin" or external ego, especially in early, regressive, or trauma-focused work. Online therapy may limit the analyst's capacity to co-regulate due to the absence of touch, a limited gaze, and delayed or filtered responses.

In summary, Tronick's Still Face experiment shows that emotional development is bodily and relational, not merely symbolic or verbal. In psychoanalysis, especially online, this raises key tensions: How can the analyst contain, attune, and co-regulate without touch, gaze, or embodied presence? How can symbolic processes compensate for these missing elements, or do they expose a gap in our theory? Jessica Benjamin (1995) draws on Tronick to develop ideas of intersubjectivity, mutual recognition, and "doer/done-to" dynamics, emphasizing the importance of mutual regulation in therapy. Daniel Stern (1985) and Beebe et al. (2002) build on similar principles, showing how *moment-to-moment nonverbal cues* shape the therapeutic alliance. Alessandra Lemma (2020) and Pat Ogden & Bonnie Goldstein (2020) warn that online therapy may fail to replicate these micro-attunements unless therapists become explicitly mindful of the missing body.

Implications for Online Psychoanalysis

From the above findings, we can conclude that there are several risks in online psychoanalysis:

- The therapist's neutral face on video may unintentionally resemble the "still face," triggering anxiety or re-enactments of early mis-attunement.
- The absence of the body may impede patients with early developmental trauma who rely on nonverbal cues for containment.
- Sensory deprivation (no touch, no physical space) might be especially challenging for borderline or psychotic structures and for patients with somatic dissociation or early relational trauma.

On the other hand, several potentials also emerge from the findings:

- The screen itself can become a transitional object or container for projection.
- Some patients feel freer to express painful or shameful material in the disembodied setting.
- The absence of physicality may amplify symbolic processes, similar to the couch setup in classical psychoanalysis.

Practically Speaking: The Impact on Neutrality and Abstinence

- *Physical setting*: In online psychotherapy, we lose the physical setting. There is no couch, no shared room, and no embodied silence. The disembodied interface changes how the analyst's neutrality is perceived. The analyst's physical absence may amplify the sense of psychic distance, or reduce it, depending on how the medium is experienced.
- *Visual presence* (or lack of it): Some online sessions are audio-only (resembling the couch setup), others use video. In video, the analyst's face is visible, which may reduce the neutrality that abstinence depends on, unless managed carefully.
- *Intrusion of the patient's environment*: The analytic "frame" is co-constructed across settings. The patient may lie on a bed, sit in a car, or be interrupted by real-life distractions. This blurs boundaries and complicates the implementation of abstinence (unless the patient is instructed to take responsibility for creating a safe holding environment with clear boundaries).
- *Maintaining abstinence online*: The analyst refrains from self-disclosure, emotional reassurance, or technical chitchat, as they would in-person. One clear advantage in the online setting is that there is no way to violate the physical boundaries of the patient and include inappropriate touch. Since the number and frequency of sexual boundary crossings in psychoanalytic setting is surprisingly high (see Gabbard, 1994), online psychotherapy reduces these unethical cases dramatically. Neutrality is preserved in tone, timing, and interpretation, though not necessarily in physical posture. Boundaries around session timing, responsiveness to emails/messages, and technical containment (e.g., using secure platforms) uphold the analytic frame.

Modifications, Creative Solutions, and Clinical Sensitivity

In general, staying within the strict and rigid frame of reference of the classical psychoanalytic approach is less recommended online, since it might increase alienation and mis-attunement.

Technological empathy (e.g., brief acknowledgment of a glitch or distress from disconnection) may be necessary and not considered a violation of abstinence if done mindfully. The relational/intersubjective model is a preferred approach to online psychoanalysis. In some traumatized or narcissistically injured patients, limited responsiveness or attunement may be therapeutically necessary even online, as argued in contemporary relational psychoanalysis.

As Weinberg et al. (2023) recommended, using creative solutions can reduce the impact of the disembodied environment online. Below are a few examples of how to compensate for the missing body:

1 The therapist can invite the patient to report their body sensations. For example, when the patient reports that they feel anxious, the therapist can ask: Where is it located in your body? What body sensations tell you that you are anxious (accelerated heartbeat, sweating)?
2 The therapist can use their tone of voice, direct the patient how to breathe, or verbalize some body functions in order to regulate a dysregulated patient. As an example, here is a possible script: "You seem overwhelmed with emotions. Listen to my voice [the therapist lowers his tone and speaks softly], breathe in … and breathe out [pause]. We can breathe in and out together. You might not be aware of it because of the screen, but I look at you now. I see you and hold you in my gaze." This kind of intervention can be quite helpful with traumatized patients having flashbacks, or any patient who becomes dysregulated online.
3 Use "body-oriented metaphorical language." For example, following an intervention, the therapist can ask: "How did my words TOUCH you?" The following is a vignette from an analytic group session: *One of the group members usually took the role of the "justice fighter," always taking care of others and fighting for any racial or gender injustice, showing her strength and not allowing her vulnerably to come up. One day, she had a terrible back ache that forced her to lie in bed immobile. She could not even drive to the doctor. She reported that this awful situation changed the power dynamics with her*

partner, since usually she was taking care of her partner, who was dependent on her. Now her partner became the one who took care of her. Exploring what might have been the psychological factors that led to her back pain, she understood that she burdened herself with other people's trouble and never allowed herself to rely on others. She became sad and when the therapist asked where the sadness is located in her body, she reported that she felt her tears stuck in her throat. The group therapist said: "We failed in lending you our shoulder to cry on" (using a bodily oriented language). This sentence released the tears, and she sobbed. Afterwards, she reported how her crying made her feel much better physically.

4 Although half of the body is missing from the screen, thus depriving the therapist of noticing leg fidgeting or other movements below the chest, the face is much bigger online than when seen in the office (except for classical analysis, using the couch). We can train ourselves to identify facial expressions more easily than when in-person and explore their meaning with the patient.

Since the above techniques can compensate for the lack of the body to an extent, but never fully replace the body-to-body interactions, I recommend meeting in person from time to time with the patient if possible. The online format should not replace the meeting in the office totally.

Clinical Insights and Emerging Views

Alessandra Lemma is one of the leading contemporary psychoanalysts grappling with how digital technology reshapes psychoanalytic practice. Across her works, especially *The Digital Age on the Couch* (2017) and *Psychoanalysis in Times of Technoculture* (2020), she explores the psychological and clinical implications of screen-mediated therapy, with a focus on the embodied presence of both patient and analyst. In her first book, Lemma (2017) highlights that online analysis offers new "screen transference" phenomena, where the analyst's image or absence onscreen becomes a canvas for projection, which can maintain abstinence in a different modality. Lemma examines how technology-mediated interactions (such as social media, virtual reality, or online therapy) affect identity formation, embodiment, and the psychoanalytic frame. She emphasizes the paradox of digital space: It feels intimate and disinhibiting yet remains fundamentally disembodied and distorting. She introduces the idea that the screen itself becomes a "psychic surface," a new canvas for transference projections. Patients may relate to the screen as a mirror, a wall, or even as maternal skin, each shaping the analytic process in distinct ways. The analyst's body in in-person work serves as a symbolic anchor, a physical presence that silently contains the patient's projections, affects, and desires. In online analysis, the analyst's body is partially or fully absent, and this undermines the symbolic function of the body as a container or boundary. Lemma warns that this absence risks regressive enactments, especially with patients who rely on sensorimotor cues to maintain psychic coherence (e.g., early trauma, borderline pathology).

In her second book (2020), Lemma deepens her exploration of how digital technologies mediate subjectivity, not just communication. She focuses on how the digital modifies the experience of the body, often leading to a disconnection between self and soma (e.g., in online identities, photoshopping, which can be a symbolic cosmetic surgery, avatar use, or selfies). She argues that analysts must be alert to how technoculture devalues the body, promoting disembodied or idealized virtual selves. The analytic setting, traditionally grounded in bodily co-presence, is challenged by online work – the absence of shared space weakens the containing function of the therapeutic frame. Nonetheless, Lemma does not reject online work. She proposes that, with awareness, the screen can support symbolic processes, provided the analyst is attuned to what's being projected into or withheld from the virtual field.

Gabriel Trop (2021) notes that the absence of physical cues may intensify symbolic thinking and internalization, sometimes deepening analytic work. Some analysts argue for a redefinition of abstinence: Not merely as withholding, but as creating space for the patient's psychic work, even within a technologically mediated frame.

Chapter 4

Practical Considerations

Legal and Ethical Issues

Before starting their first online session, psychotherapists should be aware and become knowledgeable about the legal requirements in their country regarding online therapy. Conducting psychotherapy online in the United States involves several legal and ethical considerations. Haberstroh et al. (2014) summarize these requirements. Below are some key points.

Legal Issues

1. *Licensure*: In the United States, therapists must be licensed in the state where the client is located at the time of the session. However, the Psychology Interjurisdictional Compact (PSYPACT) is an agreement that facilitates the practice of psychology across state lines in the United States. It allows licensed psychologists to conduct teletherapy in 26 states as of 2024.
2. *Informed consent*: Therapists must obtain informed consent from clients, explaining the nature of online therapy, its potential risks, and its benefits.
3. *Confidentiality*: Ensuring the confidentiality of client information is crucial. Therapists must use secure, encrypted communication platforms to protect client data. In the United States, the platform the therapist uses should be Health Insurance Portability and Accountability Act (HIPAA) compliant.

DOI: 10.4324/9781003503514-4

4 *Emergency protocols*: Therapists need to have clear protocols for handling emergencies, as they may not be able to provide immediate assistance in a crisis. Before starting therapy, they should be acquainted with emergency services at the location of the client.

Ethical Issues

1 *Competence*: Therapists must be competent in using the technology required for online therapy and understand its limitations.
2 *Boundaries*: Maintaining professional boundaries can be more challenging online. Therapists must be vigilant about setting and maintaining these boundaries. For psychodynamic therapists, maintaining boundaries is common practice; however, as mentioned in previous chapters, the online setting provides more challenges since the setting is not determined solely by the therapist, thus the patients should be instructed how to maintain boundaries as well.
3 *Privacy and security*: Protecting client privacy and ensuring the security of online communications are paramount. In addition to instructing the patients to connect from a private environment, as mentioned above, this includes using secure platforms and being aware of potential security threats.
4 *Cultural sensitivity*: Therapists must be sensitive to cultural differences that may affect the therapeutic relationship and the client's comfort with online therapy. This requirement becomes even more important online since the online setting provides more opportunities for treating patients from different countries and different cultures.

Technical and Administrative Considerations

Shall We Use the Couch?

As strange as it sounds, for psychoanalysts who use the couch daily in their practice, the shift to online psychotherapy is supposed to feel more natural since they do not rely on eye-to-eye contact when the analysand lies on the couch. Surprisingly,

Freudian psychoanalysts from the "old school" express more objections to moving online (e.g., Russell, 2015), perhaps because they hold a conservative approach that does not easily adjust itself to changes. We will discuss these resistances (both of clients and therapists) in depth in the next chapter.

Behind the question of whether to continue using the couch when shifting to online psychoanalysis lies the dilemma of how much we should stick to the same conservative techniques. I do not think that any psychoanalyst argues that the analysand should lie on the couch in front of the computer, but many psychoanalysts argue that the change of setting does not allow for "real" psychoanalysis to occur.

Gotti (2024) claims that online therapy changes the traditional psychoanalytic setting, moving it from the therapist's office to a virtual space. This shift requires a rethinking of how the therapeutic environment is structured and maintained. It emphasizes the need for a comprehensive theoretical, technical, and clinical reflection specific to each case when conducting online therapy. Treating online therapy as merely a relocation of in-person sessions can lead to misunderstandings about the depth and nature of the therapeutic connection.

The Analyst's Internal Setting

While discussing the classical analytic setting and its function in Chapter 2, we referred to the analytic contract, which includes outside realistic components and the negotiation of boundaries. But what about the analyst's internal setting? Lemma (2017) noted that the therapist's internal setting provides an important anchor as it orients the therapist to the patient's communications. She goes further to say that "it is what distinguishes an analytic therapist from any other" (p. 84). What happens, then, to the analyst's internal setting online? How do we prepare ourselves as therapists for an online setting in a way that maximizes our orientation to our patients' communications?

The fact that the analyst sits in front of the computer, sometimes at home, provides a lot of opportunities for disruption and disconnection. Glancing at iPhone notifications, reading an email on the computer while listening to the patient, being distracted by looking at one's self-image during the session, daydreaming simply because the two-dimensional figure on the screen does not alert us that we are conversing with a "real" person – all these are normal temptations when conducting online sessions. When preparing themselves for online therapy, analytic therapists should, therefore, prepare themselves physically and mentally. Physically this includes dressing properly and professionally, just as the therapist dresses for in-person meetings. Mentally, the therapist should remain keenly focused on the client and stay emotionally present in the analytic session. There might be a need for training them to do so, just as becoming a psychodynamically oriented therapist involves training in how to listen to the patient without being distracted.

Daydreaming can be considered as reverie. Ogden (1997) describes reverie as a state of mind where the therapist allows their thoughts and feelings to flow freely, often leading to unconscious material surfacing. This process helps the therapist to connect with the patient's unconscious experiences and emotions. Ogden views reverie as a crucial tool for understanding the unconscious intersubjective dynamics between the therapist and the patient. I suggest that analysts use their being distracted online in the same way and see these distractions as part of their reverie.

Dynamic Administration and the Social Unconscious

Moving online increases the number of administrative issues the therapist must deal with: Before the sessions, the therapist needs to invest time and energy in choosing a secure and reliable teletherapy platform that complies with HIPAA regulations and ensures a stable internet connection. During the session, they must deal with many technical troubleshooting issues: Internet communication can be irritating and tiring, since it involves technical difficulties such as moments of freezing video, disruption of the internet connection, gaps between lip movements and audio, and many more disruptions. The therapists must address these technical issues promptly. In addition, there is greater need to instruct patients about boundaries and maintaining privacy, and there are more frequent disruptions of those boundaries (someone enters the patient's room, the patient is muted, comes late to sessions, etc.). After the session, there is a constant need to update software and hardware regularly and to ensure backups are in place. The therapist will spend much more time dealing with the technical and administrative issues for online meetings than for office meetings.

In the group analytic field, the term "dynamic administration" relates to the administrative issues that the group analyst deals with when conducting the group. These administrative issues have a dynamic meaning (for example, arranging the chairs in a circle creates a maternal holding environment). The same idea can be applied to online psychodynamic psychotherapy: Technical difficulties and administrative issues can acquire a dynamic meaning. For example, when the internet fails and the connection is disrupted, some patients (especially those with a traumatic background and severe attachment disorders) can perceive the disconnection as abandonment by the therapist (who serves as a maternal figure). The psychodynamic therapist should remember that technical difficulties can be associated consciously or unconsciously with deeper inner fantasies. Thus, the therapist should be sensitive to those possible meanings and relate to them or interpret them. When a patient suddenly disappears, it creates a dilemma about how to interpret it. Was it voluntary? Involuntary? It also brings to the fore technical and practical issues: What do you do if you have a technical failure? Do you call? Text? Who calls? How long do you stay online if they disappear?

Borrowing further from the group analytic literature, we can build on the social unconscious concept (Hopper and Weinberg, 2011, 2015, 2017), which should be explored in psychoanalytic therapy beyond the personal unconscious. Hopper (2001, p. 10) defines the social unconscious thus:

> The concept of the Social Unconscious refers to the existence and constraints of social, cultural and communicational arrangements of which people are unaware. Unaware, in so far as these arrangements are not perceived (not "known"), and if perceived not acknowledged ("denied"), and if

> acknowledged, not taken as problematic ("given"), and if taken as problematic, not considered with an optimal degree of detachment and objectivity.

Weinberg (2007, p. 312) claims that the Social Unconscious includes "shared anxieties, fantasies, defenses, myths, and memories."

However, Hopper (2023) claims that "The concept of the social unconscious refers to the social, cultural, communicational, and *technological* 'arrangements' of which people are unaware" (p. 2, italics mine). This is an important addition to the dimensions that should be considered when dealing with the social unconscious. So far it has included dimensions such as norms, values, gender, communication, and relations. Now it is expanded to include the technological dimension (just as for Karl Marx, technology exemplifies the interaction between human beings and nature). This dimension evokes associations and unconscious fantasies, adding a technological dimension to the social unconscious. We might even relate to this aspect as "the internet unconscious."

Turkle et al. (2017) say: "Technology creates a new state of the self, itself. Online intimacies are real but operate with new dynamics" (p. 242). Weinberg (2014) argued that online relationships involve a different kind of intimacy and termed it *E-ntimacy*. It does not embody the kind of "into-me-you-see" that Hollywood movies glorify, which relies on self-disclosure and privacy. Online E-ntimacy is more like the kind of intimacy that develops in large groups and is based on an atmosphere of cohesion, "we-ness," and belonging.

The difficult question is when to interpret technology failures and when to relate to them concretely. When the patient comes late to an online meeting, claiming that they have trouble connecting to the internet, is it an example of resistance that should be interpreted? In fact, this question is not unique to online meetings. The same dilemma occurs when the patient explains his lateness to an in-person meeting by saying that there was a traffic jam. The decision depends on the frequency of these behaviors, other signs of resistance, and how beneficial it would be in this stage of therapy to interpret it.

The following is an example of how a technical issue revealed a psychological dynamic beyond it. *During a session, the patient commented on making the therapist's image bigger on his screen.*

The therapist became curious and wanted to understand more. Technically, it seemed as if the patient shifted from the gallery view on Zoom, in which both partners show side by side with the same size, to speaker view, in which the therapist is shown in the center, much bigger, and the picture of the patient is much smaller. The therapist wanted to understand the motivation behind this act. This led to a discussion that revealed the idealization of the therapist by the patient (making him "bigger"), and how the patient belittles himself by using this psychological mechanism.

Another example of using technology in the service of psychological processes comes from a long-term open-ended online group session conducted by two co-leaders, one male and one female. *In this session, one of the group members terminated her membership in the group after three years of participation, announcing it several weeks beforehand. While discussing her long journey and what she gained during the group meetings, the member mentioned that she always arranged the pictures of the group members on the screen (an option available on the Zoom application) so that the two group leaders would show at the top of the screen with her picture between them. Group members were curious about her motivation, and she explained that she felt held by the conductors. She continued to describe the maternal nurturing holding she felt from the female conductor and how she had wanted to be close to the male conductor, but after allowing it, she became frightened and withdrew. As time passed, she felt that she could trust the male conductor more and that he would not hurt her.* In this example, exploring technical issues enriched the discussion with glimpses of transferences and relational issues.

Shifting from the In-Person to the Online Setting

The shift from meeting face-to-face in the office to seeing patients online provides a rare opportunity to understand the specific psychodynamics involved in teletherapy. I am not referring to the forced, dramatic, hasty shift that occurred at the beginning of 2020 around the world due to the pandemic, but to an organized, well-planned, prepared-in-advance decision some psychotherapists made to move online. Here is an interesting example from my practice when I decided to make this move.

The patient was a well-established businessman who came to therapy because of depression that was triggered by a difficult sociopolitical atmosphere, which harmed his business. He was involved with the local politics and used to feel that he had control over political issues and could exert his power, have an influence, and make a difference. For many sessions, he complained about politics, expressed his irritation and anger over the faulty decisions of the politicians, and described his business empire, trying to impress the therapist with his power. It was very difficult to direct him to talk about his personal issues and stop intellectualizing. The therapist used a self-psychology empathic attitude and mainly interpreted the need for mirroring and the difficulty in feeling helpless. From time to time, this patient talked about his kids or his parents, but, although he was married, he never mentioned his relationship with his wife.

Then the therapist (me) decided to quit his physical office and move to online sessions only. I announced well in advance and welcomed any emotional response. The patient felt sad, said that he would miss the in-person closeness, but understood the reasons and did not see it as problematic. Several weeks before the scheduled move to online meetings, he suddenly started talking about his diminished sexual desire and revealed a conflict around intimate issues with his wife. This was a very abrupt change from his usual style and non-personal discussion.

There are many ways to understand this shift, and we explored many aspects, but the relevant interesting aspect is how it was connected to the change in the setting. Apparently, the patient felt that this was his last chance to bring intimate issues to the meetings since he was not sure that he would feel comfortable discussing them in online meetings. However, when we eventually met online, he said that in a weird way he felt closer since he saw my head bigger and closer. He continued to bring personal and intimate issues to the online sessions.

Online Rupture and Repair

Rupture and repair became an important issue in psychodynamic literature in recent decades. (Larsson et al., 2018; Miller-Bottome et al., 2019; Humer et al., 2021; Dolev-Amit et al., 2020).

Ruptures create "a deterioration in the therapeutic alliance, manifested by a disagreement between the patient and therapist on treatment goals, a lack of collaboration on therapeutic tasks, or a strain in their emotional bond" (Eubanks et al., 2018, p. 508). Ruptures in the therapeutic alliance are common. If left unresolved, they can lead patients to drop out, among other poor outcomes.

Since human beings are prone to making mistakes, there will always be some ruptures in the therapeutic alliance. This means that the focus in therapeutic relationships should shift from being perfect and trying to prevent mistakes to repairing mistakes when they happen. Focusing on repairing mistakes and empathic failures in therapy can deeply affect the therapeutic process, more than intellectual interpretations, since they touch a deep unconscious wish that our early caregivers acknowledge and apologize for their unattuned responses from our childhood.

Repairing therapeutic ruptures is an important process that is relevant for practitioners of all theoretical orientations, but especially for psychodynamic practitioners who hold self-psychological and relational approaches. According to those approaches, the therapist/analyst should take into account their unconscious processes that affect the therapeutic interventions. The reactions of the patient do not always originate from projective "non-real" transference responses. Some of them might be responses to real empathic failures created by the therapist. Safran and Muran (2000) identified two types of alliance ruptures: Withdrawal and confrontation. Withdrawal ruptures refer to those instances when the client responds to difficulties, misunderstandings, or disagreements in the therapeutic relationship by moving *away from* the therapist, either by falling silent and offering minimal responses to questions, or by denying an aspect of his or her experience. By contrast, a confrontation rupture is characterized by the client moving *against* the therapist, expressing anger or dissatisfaction with the therapist or treatment.

Surely, withdrawal ruptures are more difficult for the therapist to identify, and in online therapy they are even more difficult to see. Usually, the therapist relies on nonverbal signs for withdrawal responses to identify this kind of rupture. The lack of somatic queues and the absence of body-to-body interactions in the online setting make it difficult for the therapist to sense the withdrawal of the patient and they must rely on other hints, such as more silence, etc. This means that the online psychodynamic therapist should pay special attention to their countertransference reactions and consider the possibility that some of those reactions are an unconscious response to the withdrawal of the patient. Dolev-Amit, Leibovich & Zilcha-Mano (2020) provide detailed guidelines for therapists on how supportive techniques developed in traditional face-to-face treatment can be effectively used in telepsychotherapy to resolve alliance ruptures. As mentioned above, they too point out that confrontation ruptures (characterized by overt expression of anger and dissatisfaction) are easier to detect both online and offline, but withdrawal ruptures (moving away from the therapist through avoidance or detached behavior) that can go unnoticed by therapists in face-to-face treatment, are even more challenging in telepsychotherapy. This is due to both the disembodied environment and the technical failures. They suggest that therapists create an appropriate setting and basic technical conditions and pay greater attention to the nuances of the patient's in-session behavior.

Muran et al. (2022) referred to the Critical-Cultural-Relational Model that emphasizes the role of cultural and relational factors in alliance ruptures and repairs. The model suggests that addressing these factors can lead to more effective resolution of ruptures. They also suggest that in short-term psychodynamic psychotherapy, it is important to address ruptures early in the therapeutic process to prevent dropout and improve treatment outcomes.

Chapter 5

Transference, Countertransference, and Resistance Online

Definition of the Terms

Transference and countertransference are fundamental concepts in psychoanalytic psychotherapy. They refer to unconscious emotional responses that occur within the therapeutic relationship. Freud introduced the concepts of transference and resistance as central to the therapeutic process. We will first define these concepts and then describe their online application. Some of these concepts changed and developed along the history of psychoanalysis, and we should clarify to which definition of the concept we refer. For example, countertransference was considered problematic in the conservative classical psychanalytic approach, however, Paula Heimann (1950) was one of the pioneers who began to see countertransference differently. She argued that countertransference could provide valuable insights into the patient's unconscious. Harris (2005) reviews the evolution of transference and countertransference matrices through major psychoanalytic schools and theories.

Transference

Transference is the unconscious redirection of feelings and attitudes from important figures in the patient's past onto the therapist. It is not just about seeing the therapist as a parental figure or a past lover. It is about the deep-seated emotional baggage getting unpacked in the therapy room. These feelings can be positive or

DOI: 10.4324/9781003503514-5

negative and often manifest as intense emotional reactions, such as love, hate, anger, or dependence. By understanding these unconscious projections, therapists can gain valuable insights into the patient's inner world and past relationships. It is crucial for uncovering unresolved conflicts and working through them.

Kohut (1971) expanded on the concept of transference by introducing the idea of self-object transferences. He viewed transference as a reflection of the patient's unmet developmental needs. The difference between the classical transference concept and the self-psychological one can go unnoticed at first, but it is quite crucial: While classical transference reactions relate to the unconscious repetition of early object relations, in the self-psychological frame of reference, the patient transfers what they lack, their wished-for needs. These needs, Kohut argued, were rooted in missing early childhood experiences, particularly the unfulfilled need for empathy and mirroring. He identified three main types of transferences: Mirror transference (seeking validation and admiration), idealizing transference (seeking guidance and support), and twinship transference (seeking a sense of belonging and connection).

Countertransference

Countertransference refers to the therapist's unconscious emotional reactions to the patient, influenced by the therapist's own background and personal history. These reactions can be triggered by the patient's transference, the therapist's own unresolved issues, or a combination of both. Therapists need to be aware of their own countertransference reactions, as they can impact the therapeutic relationship and hinder the therapeutic process. Properly managed, countertransference can be a powerful tool for understanding the patient's experience, but if it goes unchecked, it can distort the therapist's objectivity.

Winnicott distinguishes between the concepts of objective and subjective countertransference in psychoanalytic practice:

- *Objective countertransference*: Refers to the therapist's emotional response that mirrors the patient's feelings and experiences from their past relationships. It is seen as a repetition of

the patient's emotional history, induced by the patient's behavior and communication in therapy. It is assumed that most therapists would respond this way to the patient. For example, patients who complain all the time and lack the ability to feel gratitude can be irritating to many therapists. Winnicott viewed this as a valuable tool for understanding the patient's internal world and past relational patterns (see Geltner, 2006).
- *Subjective countertransference*: This involves the therapist's personal, unconscious reactions to the patient, influenced by the therapist's own background and unresolved conflicts. Unlike objective countertransference, subjective countertransference can potentially interfere with the therapeutic process if not properly managed.

Winnicott's distinction helps therapists differentiate between their own personal reactions and the patient's emotional projections, allowing for more effective therapeutic interventions.

The concepts of transference and countertransference are important because they help the therapist understand the patient's dynamics: By examining transference, therapists can gain insight into the patient's unresolved conflicts and attachment patterns. Understanding these processes can also guide therapeutic intervention: Therapists can use transference as a tool for exploration and interpretation, helping patients to understand their unconscious motivations and behaviors. They can also increase the self-awareness of the therapist: Recognizing and managing countertransference is essential for maintaining objectivity and providing effective therapy. The idea of objective countertransference further helps the therapist to get in touch with the patient's unconscious dynamics.

Before we move to exploring these concepts in online therapy, I would like to mention the way that relationally oriented psychodynamic therapists relate to these processes: In these approaches (Greenberg and Mitchell, 1983; Aron, 1996), it is taken for granted that the therapist has an unconscious too. Relational psychoanalysis emphasizes that both the patient and therapist co-create the therapeutic experience. Thus, we cannot distinguish between countertransference and transference processes. Countertransference is actually the transference of the therapist. The therapist's countertransference is seen as a two-way street, where the therapist's own internal world interacts with the patient's projections, creating a unique therapeutic dynamic. Therefore, relational therapists talk about the transference-countertransference matrix, since the processes cannot be separated.

While both transference and countertransference can be challenging, they can also be powerful tools for therapeutic growth and change. By understanding and utilizing these concepts, psychotherapists can create a safe and supportive environment for their patients to explore their deepest emotions and work toward healing.

Transference and Countertransference in the Online Setting

Video therapy introduces several types of transference and countertransference relations. My experience shows that many transference reactions exist in cyberspace, in the same way that they exist in our office. For example, from the classical, traditional point of view, the therapist can be perceived as a strict parental figure online, just as the patient projects on the therapist their strict and rigid mother or father when meeting in-person. Can the reader identify whether the following short vignette occurred in the office or online?

The patient was regularly late to the sessions. The psychotherapist suggested exploring the reasons behind this continuous lateness. In response, the patient complained that the therapist was critical of him and angry with him. The patient wondered whether the therapist felt disrespected. Since the therapist did not sense any anger and did not think that the patient's lateness was disrespectful, he became curious about the source of these perceptions. Deep exploration revealed that the patient's father was very critical of him and scolded him many times for not being respectful enough toward his father. It sounded as if the patient projected his rigid and narcissistic father onto the therapist.

Did you guess that this event occurred online?

In addition to the classical transference phenomena, online psychotherapy provides opportunities for self-object transference processes, as described in the self-psychological frame of reference. Agar (2020) focuses on Kohut's self-psychological transferences and argues that both the choice of video therapy by the therapist and patient, and their co-presence onscreen, have meaning at the transferential and countertransferential level, gaining a quality of partnership, twinship, and merging. The online therapist becomes a vaguer figure than the therapist in the office, making them less known (at least in the first stages of therapy), allowing for more projections of inner object relations and world of fantasy. Agar adds that the absence of the physical therapy room leads to blurring the boundary between the therapist as an object and the therapist as a therapeutic function. Video therapy has qualities that encourage the patient to feel momentarily that they are "creating" the therapist, allowing childhood omnipotence fantasies to surface in therapy. All these factors expedite internalization of the therapeutic functions and create a symbolic continuity of therapeutic relationship between sessions.

Agar (2020) brings a case that exemplifies how the therapist and the patient online create a mutual relationship, thus participating in the transference-countertransference matrix as described in the relational frame of reference. *For the online session she (the therapist, Agar) wore a new outfit, of which she was extremely fond, and the patient mistook it for pajamas. The therapist was surprised but later understood that the upper part, which was the only one shown on the screen, can look like pajamas.* The patient has learned about the therapist's subjectivity seeing the therapist's surprised reaction and hearing her protest that it was not pajamas but a smart outfit. The patient experienced mutuality and felt her impact on the therapist as the therapist commented that she could understand through the patient how not everyone would consider that outfit to be smart.

However, teletherapy can also lead to unique transference reactions not seen with in-person therapy. The elements that stimulate these reactions online are often elements related to the medium's technical limitations and are influenced by the virtual environment and the therapist's background (Eichenberger & Boswell, 2024). Psychotherapists should be mindful of how the teletherapy frame affects transference and therapeutic relationships and adapt their approach accordingly. The virtual nature of teletherapy offers "an additional dimension of irreality to the symbolic and imagined transference relationship" (Eichenberger & Boswell, 2024, p. 18) and can affect interpersonal dynamics between psychotherapist and patient. However, this change need not be seen as a hindrance to therapy. Instead, transference in teletherapy can be viewed as a meaningful facet of treatment to understand. Additionally, teletherapy may lead to a "safety of distance," allowing access to fantasies and topics that may not arise during in-person therapy. Matheson and Kegerreis (2023) also found that working online offered different and exciting opportunities for therapy, including the unconscious processes that are central to the psychodynamic modality.

The following is an example of a countertransference reaction unique to the online setting and related to the technological component. *In an online group setting, one of the members criticized the group analysts, saying that he was "sharp" with her. The group conductor welcomed her criticism and suggested exploring her feelings and the group's reactions. She started to talk and suddenly became quiet. The group analyst wondered what had happened and noticed that she was muted. He asked her why she muted herself, and she opened her microphone and claimed that it wasn't her who muted herself. To his surprise and dismay, the conductor suddenly understood that his finger inadvertently clicked on her microphone's icon and muted her. This action was made unconsciously, without even noticing, as if his body had its own will. He acknowledged that probably his unconscious "tricked" him to reveal his countertransference, a denied part of his feelings.*

Braude et al. (2023) conducted qualitative interviews with 16 Australian psychologists and found that the type of countertransference reactions toward existing clients was consistent across both face-to-face and online meetings; This finding is important in reassuring us that when we work online we still have the same emotional reactions toward our patients. In order to conduct a productive psychoanalytic session in cyberspace, we should be aware that our countertransference might be similar to the one we have in-person. However, in the above-cited research, the felt intensity of countertransference reactions was reduced.

Psychologists reported an increased hesitance to work with intense emotions during telepsychotherapy sessions and felt increased pressure to work harder during online sessions when compared to face-to-face meetings. Exposure to their clients' personal and home environments during telepsychotherapy sessions elicited several novel reactions toward their clients.

Hiding Self-View?

An example of how the medium's technical features influence dynamic processes, including transference and counter-transference, is the fact that, in online communication, the therapist and the patient see their own image on the screen. Indeed, they can use the "hide self-view" option but doing this creates a different situation than in the in-person meeting (for example, the patient who hides self-view might not notice that his face is not fully seen on the screen). The mirror function is embedded in the actual communicative medium of Zoom virtual psychotherapy, which means that the screen embodies a sense of being in the world (Dudai & Metzl, 2024). It can offer a projective and transferential space, crucial to the interpersonal relational dialogue in which we see one another as subjects. Dudai & Metzl (2024) argue that the unique quality of Zoom psychotherapy, by which the ability to dismantle the components of the image (using only sound without video), represents the transference, a psychic retreat into darkness. This dyadic interaction via screen virtuality creates a space to explore "who is seeing" as well as experiences of "seeing and being seen."

Bar (2023) suggested that when patients see themselves on the screen through their "self-view," they encounter disconnected aspects of themselves that are less accessible to them or that they are less in touch with and therefore are experienced as "not me." It *is* the "me," but it is the presentation of the less sparkling, glamorous, attractive, or familiar self-state. This "otherness" can be used as an ongoing simulation, and the high emotional arousal that it brings to the surface can be used as an opportunity for growth. As such, virtual space is an opportunity to expand the self and accept the non-self as part of the self. In virtual work, for both the therapist and the client, the participating self is experienced as a subjective self, i.e., "me," while the onscreen self is newly experienced as an object and therefore as an alien and isolated, "not me."

Usually, when patients hide their self-view, it is unnoticed by the therapist. However, sometimes this fact is revealed either spontaneously by the patient mentioning it, or when it seems that the patient is unaware that their face is not seen fully on the screen. The therapist might ask the patient what is happening, and the patient's response can reveal that they hid their self-view. This disclosure can lead to an in-depth exploration of the reasons for this hiding. Some patients do not like the way they look, and exploration of this theme can bring to the front questions of body image, etc.

The Computer as an Extension of the Self

Among other interesting phenomena when working online, we should pay attention to the relevant psychological idea that the computer is experienced as an extension of the patient's and therapist's body and self. In *The Second Self* (2005), Turkle describes how people react strongly to a computer crash, as if their computer is expected to function as a natural part of the user's body. The computer is perceived not as a "tool," but as part of our social and psychological lives. When the internet fails and the online session crashes, we feel very frustrated. Most of the time we tend to "blame" the other side first for the failure and suspect that their internet connection is weak. In a therapy session, this can become part of the transference-countertransference matrix. It can be overt when the therapist overtly tells the client that their internet failed, or covert when the thought is kept inside, but still affects the therapist's attitude toward the patient.

In summary, transference and countertransference show themselves in online work, just as they do in our office. However, in addition to the classical transference reactions, in which the patient projects their early caregivers onto the therapist, and the self-object transference, in which the patient transfers what was absent in the original attitude of the caregivers, there are unique transferences online that stem from the technological features of the media.

Resistance

Resistance, Freud argued, is a defense mechanism employed by the ego to protect the unconscious from anxiety-provoking thoughts and feelings. In psychoanalytic psychotherapy, resistance refers to the unconscious mechanisms that prevent individuals from bringing repressed thoughts, feelings, or drives into conscious awareness. Freud first identified resistance as patients' uncooperative behaviors during therapy sessions. He believed that these behaviors were attempts to avoid confronting distressing unconscious material.

Resistance is seen as a defense mechanism that protects the individual from experiencing psychological pain. It can manifest in various ways, such as missing sessions, changing the subject, or being overly intellectual. Overcoming resistance is a key part of the therapeutic process, as it allows for the integration of repressed material into consciousness, leading to greater self-awareness and psychological healing.

Resistance to/in Online Therapy

As noted in the section about transference and countertransference, resistance to analytic work can take the same shape online as it does in-person. Anxiety-provoking repressed thoughts and feelings can threaten patients in online meetings as well, so we can anticipate that defense mechanisms will show up and that resistance emerges. In online therapy, resistance can manifest in both overt and subtle ways, influenced by the medium's inherent characteristics. While extensively studied in traditional face-to-face therapy, resistance can manifest differently in the virtual environment due to the distinct dynamics of online communication.

Some common manifestations include the following.

1 *Avoidance behaviors*: Clients may avoid logging into sessions, cancel appointments frequently, or delay responding to messages in asynchronous modalities. These behaviors can reflect a reluctance to engage with the therapeutic process or address challenging issues.

2 *Technological excuses*: The virtual nature of online therapy offers opportunities for resistance to be framed as technical difficulties. For example, clients might claim poor internet connectivity, malfunctioning devices, or software issues to avoid engaging in sessions.
3 *Superficial communication*: Clients may adopt a detached or superficial style of interaction, using the screen as a barrier to evade deeper emotional exploration. This can include over-reliance on humor, vagueness in discussing personal issues, or focusing excessively on external topics unrelated to therapy.
4 *Hypercontrol of the environment*: Unlike in traditional therapy settings, clients have greater control over their surroundings in online therapy. Resistance might manifest as distractions in the environment, such as having other individuals present, multi-tasking during sessions, or choosing settings that limit privacy.

The causes of psychological resistance in online therapy are multifaceted and often rooted in a combination of personal, relational, and technological factors:

1 *Fear of vulnerability*: The physical distance in online therapy may amplify fears of vulnerability, as clients might question the therapist's ability to truly "see" and understand them in a virtual context.
2 *Lack of familiarity with the medium*: Clients who are unfamiliar or uncomfortable with digital platforms may experience heightened anxiety or skepticism about the therapeutic process, leading to resistance.
3 *Perceived anonymity*: The virtual format can create a sense of anonymity, which, while initially disinhibiting, may also encourage resistance by reducing accountability.
4 *Reduced nonverbal cues*: The lack of physical presence and reduced access to nonverbal cues can hinder the therapeutic alliance, making it easier for clients to disengage or withhold emotional expression.

The reader should be aware that sometimes the patient can use the technological aspects, or even the fact that the therapy is conducted online, as an excuse to drop out of therapy. While online therapy is not suitable for everyone, patients might use this argument as a way of avoiding deeper exploration of themselves. It is not easy to decide when it is a justified reason for ending the online sessions, and when it is just an excuse and should be considered as resistance.

Below is a relevant case vignette from a group analytic group.[1]

Karen joined an online process group led by the author after participating in a two-day face-to-face process group led by the author at a group therapy conference. In that workshop, she was very impressed by the group leader's skills and felt that he understood her deeply. She perceived him as giving her special attention and being very attuned to her. However, a few months after she had joined the weekly online group, she felt very disappointed. She did not feel as special as she felt in the intensive face-to-face group at the conference, and she thought that she did not draw the leader's attention as she expected. She said something about losing his attention in the group, but the topic was not explored much further. A few weeks later she wrote an e-mail to the group leader, letting him know that she was considering leaving the group. She blamed it on the fact that it was an online group and that she could not build the connection she was used to creating in a group meeting in-person. She wrote that the online format did not work very well for her. She added that there was something about not being in the same physical space, at the same time, that presented a barrier to the group process for her. The group leader suggested that she bring this issue for discussion in the group, sticking to the common practice of in-person groups that everything relevant to the group process that is discussed outside the group, should be brought back to the group, especially when someone considers termination. She agreed and in the next online group session she told the group that she did not think that the online format suited her. As usual with such announcements, people's reactions varied between expressing sorrow and sadness and being irritated. They did not suggest exploring her motives further. Eventually, the group leader asked whether it meant that they agreed with her that the online modality did not allow for "real" connection. This intervention helped the discussion to deepen, and one member suggested that perhaps there are other issues that were blocking her ability to connect. The group leader reminded her how disappointed she was about not getting enough attention from him and wondered whether it was more meaningful than she had allowed herself to imagine or experience. After the conversation began to move away from this dialogue between Karen and the leader, Nina (a group member) said, "Karen, I can see that the connection between you and Haim is important to you right now, and I want you to have that. I want to do whatever I can to help you have it." Karen became tearful and was deeply touched by this sacrifice. She remembered that in her family of origin, her youngest sister always received her father's full attention, and she painfully longed for him to pay attention to her as well. She was shocked that this group "sister" of hers did not play the role she had expected. All the group members were touched by Nina's generosity. When the group leader asked Nina whether she could reflect on her motivation, Nina understood that Karen was her "sister," too, that in fact, at that point in time, Nina's father was battling the end stages of cancer, and Nina desperately wanted her own sister to receive the validation of her relationship with their father. Nina had the opportunity to realize the painful impact on herself of Nina's sister's longing to be validated by their father.

To address resistance in online therapy, therapists can employ several strategies. Building a strong therapeutic alliance is crucial, as it fosters trust and encourages clients to open up. Therapists should also be mindful of their communication style, ensuring that they are empathetic, non-judgmental, and supportive. Therapists can openly discuss the potential for resistance in online therapy, normalizing it as a common part of the therapeutic process and inviting clients to explore their feelings about the medium. Therapists should tailor interventions to suit the online format, incorporating creative approaches such as screen-sharing, guided imagery, or mindfulness exercises delivered virtually.

In addition to resistance during the online psychoanalytic process, we should pay attention to the resistance to online psychoanalysis per se. Adjusting to the new situation and understanding that telehealth is a necessary fact was not easy for many of our colleagues when the pandemic hit. Psychoanalysts claimed, "This is not psychoanalysis." In general, we can describe one of the major resistances to online psychoanalysis as following the metaphor of Magritte's famous painting "Ceci n'est pas une pipe" (French; English translation "This is not a pipe"). Although the painting does show a pipe, it is not "the real thing," as it is only a two-dimensional representation of a three-dimensional object. Accordingly, those who claim that online psychoanalysis is not *real* psychoanalysis believe that even if the online analysis resembles a meeting in-person, there is no way that it can be the same.

The attempt to force online therapy to be exactly the same as in-person therapy is futile. If we take this idea to the extreme, when moving online, therapists who use the psychoanalytic couch in their office should insist that the patient lie on the couch in front of the computer screen, which seems quite a rigid approach.

Some resistances to online therapy stem from the risk of totally losing the boundaries of the session. For example, Russell (2015) claims that "A bed is not a couch, and a car is not a consulting room" (p. 13). True, indeed. But it is easy to instruct the patient not to connect to the session from their beds or while driving. We can compare the lack of control of the boundaries online to the situation offline, where, for example, we cannot control whether patients come under the influence of substances. Others claim that the analyst cannot create the same therapeutic presence online. However, Carlino (2011) argues that presence is no longer linked to physical proximity and that psychoanalytic methods can continue to be applied to new technologically mediated settings. Geller (2023) demonstrates that therapists can establish therapeutic presence online as well. She recommends training for therapeutic presence that includes preparing for presence through intention before and during the session.

Other therapists are concerned about the risk of being distracted by emails, phone messages, etc. (for both patients and therapists). Since becoming a psychodynamically oriented therapist involves training in how to listen to the patient without being distracted, I assume that training for online psychoanalysis can teach staying focused online as well. Ogden (1997) recommends using the analyst's reverie to connect to and understand the patient's unconscious processes. Analysts can use their being distracted online the same way and see these distractions as part of their reverie. As for the patient, just as we instruct them to use free associations, bring dreams, etc., we can instruct them on how to stay focused online.

Turkle (2011) is concerned that "growing up tethered" to the internet is a major source of stress in our modern lives. She is worried that using the internet to overcome geographical distance and to avoid possible termination of therapy is encouraging immediate gratification and is against the importance of delayed gratification in patients' mature development. It might create the illusion that one can always ignore and overcome loss. However, the frustrating elements in internet connection (such as the lack of body-to-body interaction and internet connection failures) can teach the patient that not everything they wish for can be achieved online. Since all online therapies end eventually, sooner or later, the therapist has the opportunity to work on termination and loss when it comes to ending therapy at a distance.

To keep the balance, we have to acknowledge that the opposite can also be true, and that some patients and therapists might develop resistance to getting back to in-person meetings, for psychological reasons. Trub (2024) identifies several psychological forces influencing the decision to remain remote, such as guilt, anxiety about self-interest, unmourned losses, collective PTSD, and existential fears about technology replacing human interaction. She argues that therapists may be rationalizing their choice to stay remote by downplaying the limitations and potential negative impacts of online therapy. This denial could threaten the integrity of psychoanalytic practice. Trub calls for a critical examination of these trends.

Note

1 This case appears in Weinberg (2020b).

Chapter 6

Special Populations and Modalities

Introduction

While considering online psychoanalytic psychotherapy, we should take into consideration the unique challenges and benefits of conducting it with specific populations, including the impact on therapeutic alliance, engagement, and outcomes among these populations, requiring adaptations to theoretical frameworks and therapeutic techniques. In this chapter I focus on the special challenges applying online therapy to children and adolescents, as well as to couples. I also discuss conducting analytic group therapy online.

Online Psychoanalytic Therapy with Children and Adolescents

Psychoanalytic therapy with children and adolescents aims to help them understand and manage their emotions, develop healthier coping strategies, and improve their functioning and relationships. One of the primary challenges of online therapy with children and adolescents is establishing a strong therapeutic alliance (American Psychoanalytic Association). The lack of physical presence can make it more difficult for therapists to build trust and rapport with young clients. Additionally, young children may struggle with the technology required for online sessions, leading to distractions and disengagement. Despite these challenges, online therapy offers several benefits. It provides greater accessibility, allowing children and adolescents in remote or underserved areas to receive therapy.

DOI: 10.4324/9781003503514-6

Online sessions can also be more flexible, accommodating busy schedules and reducing the stigma associated with seeking mental health support, which can be crucial for adolescents who are very sensitive to their peers' opinions. For adolescents, who spend a lot of time online and are very used to connecting through the internet, online therapy may seem very natural and appealing. The virtual format can facilitate greater parental involvement when appropriate. For example, parents can join at the beginning or end of a session to discuss concerns or progress, fostering a collaborative therapeutic alliance. Adapting online therapy for younger populations should emphasize developmental, relational, and technological considerations.

Psychoanalytic therapy for children and adolescents is rooted in principles such as unconscious processes, transference, countertransference, as in any psychoanalytic approach, adding especially the role of play and symbolism. In an online setting, these principles must be adapted to accommodate the digital medium:

1 *Symbolic play in virtual spaces*: Symbolic play is a cornerstone of psychoanalytic work with children. In online therapy, therapists incorporate technology creatively, using digital tools, such as drawing apps, online games, multimedia, or shared virtual whiteboards, to facilitate exploration and expression and to create a space where symbolic expression can occur. Teleplay therapy might expose the therapist to the entire system of the child's world. For example, a child might use drawing software to depict their inner world, which can then be explored collaboratively. Adolescents might find it easier to discuss difficult topics through creative media such as shared playlists or digital storytelling.

2 *Transference and countertransference*: While transference can still emerge in online therapy, the absence of physical presence may alter its dynamics. Adolescents, in particular, may project their feelings onto the therapist's virtual persona (e.g., interpreting delays in response as disinterest). Countertransference, too, can be influenced by the medium, as therapists must be mindful of their reactions to technical difficulties or the unique stressors of remote work.

3 *The holding environment*: Winnicott's concept of the "holding environment" (1965) is crucial in psychoanalytic therapy for children and adolescents. In virtual therapy, the therapist must create an emotionally safe space for the young person despite the physical distance. This requires attentiveness to verbal and nonverbal cues, as well as ensuring a consistent and reliable online presence. The attention span of children might be shorter than that of adults, especially in an online setting, which means that shorter sessions might be needed.

Online psychoanalytic therapy with children and adolescents poses distinct challenges, including:

1 *Technological barriers*: Issues such as unstable internet connections, software malfunctions, or lack of access to devices can disrupt the therapeutic process. Younger children, in particular, may struggle to engage with technology in a therapeutic manner.
2 *Attention and engagement*: Maintaining the attention and engagement of children and adolescents online can be challenging. Unlike in-person sessions, where therapists can utilize physical space and movement to keep the child's interest, the virtual format requires more creative strategies to sustain focus. Good examples of creative strategies in working with children can be found in Keating (2023). In Keating's chapter, he brings case examples illustrating how to establish safety and trust by advocating for a private space and following the child's inner wisdom over multiple sessions.
3 *Privacy and confidentiality*: Ensuring privacy is a significant concern in online therapy, particularly when children or adolescents attend sessions from home. External interruptions, shared spaces, or parental monitoring can compromise confidentiality and affect the client's willingness to open.
4 *Developmental considerations*: Children and adolescents are at different stages of cognitive and emotional development, which affects their capacity to engage in online therapy. Younger children may have difficulty understanding the therapeutic frame in a virtual setting, while adolescents might be more comfortable but less willing to explore vulnerable emotions.

To address the challenges of online therapy, therapists can employ several strategies. Building a strong therapeutic alliance is crucial. This can be achieved through consistent communication, empathy, and active listening. Therapists should also be mindful of their communication style, ensuring that they are engaging and supportive. For detailed practice guidelines for tele-mental health with children and adolescents, see Myers et al. (2017).

Case Example

Consider the case of a 12-year-old boy referred for online psychoanalytic therapy due to anxiety and social withdrawal. In initial sessions, the therapist observed the boy's reluctance to engage verbally. Using a shared drawing app, the boy began illustrating scenes from his daily life, which opened a window into his internal world. Over time, the therapist interpreted recurring themes in the drawings, linking them to the boy's feelings of isolation and fear of rejection. The therapeutic work progressed as the boy became more comfortable discussing these emotions verbally, facilitated by the safe and creative online environment.

Online Psychoanalytic Couple Therapy

The practice of psychoanalytic couple therapy has long relied on the intimate dynamics of the therapeutic space, where partners explore unconscious patterns, transference, and relational conflicts under the guidance of a therapist. For example, Scharff and Scharff (2000) developed an object relations couple therapy that values affect, silence, body language, fantasy, dreams, and transference phenomena as necessary for reaching the unconscious to achieve insight. The object relations therapist interprets defenses against anxieties that underlie repetitive patterns of unhelpful behavior and works toward understanding. Therapists use countertransference to understand the couple's shared transference from inside their experience.

With the advent of digital technology, this modality has expanded into the virtual realm, raising questions about its efficacy, adaptability, and therapeutic alliance. Online psychoanalytic couple therapy offers both unique opportunities and challenges that merit careful exploration. For some populations (e.g. military or long-distance couples) the internet creates a wonderful opportunity to work at problems in their relationships. Bagnini (2015), a psychodynamic couple therapist, calls the technology involved in videoconferencing a "fourth object" in the treatment of the couple. Both the couple and the therapist are sensitive to the added burden of depending on the "technology mother" that can create opportunity but can also let the threesome down. Let us examine the theoretical foundations, practical adaptations, and potential limitations of conducting psychoanalytic couple therapy in an online setting.

1. *Transference and countertransference*: The couple's dynamics often mirror unresolved conflicts from their individual pasts. Online therapy retains the potential for these projections but alters their expression due to the digital medium. For instance, the absence of physical presence may amplify or dilute transference phenomena.
2. *The holding environment*: Drawing from Winnicott's concept of the "holding environment" (1965), the therapist creates a safe space for partners to explore vulnerabilities. Online platforms challenge the creation of such an environment, as factors such as unstable internet connections or distractions in the home setting can disrupt the therapeutic frame.
3. *Unconscious communication*: Nonverbal cues such as body language and subtle facial expressions are essential in psychoanalytic therapy. While online therapy provides visual contact, it often limits the therapist's ability to fully observe and interpret these cues.

To maintain the efficacy of psychoanalytic couple therapy in a virtual format, therapists must adapt their practices to the unique characteristics of the online medium. Key adaptations include:

1. *Technological considerations*: Therapists must ensure the use of secure, reliable videoconferencing platforms that prioritize privacy and confidentiality. Clear guidelines about technical issues, such as how to handle disconnections, should be established at the outset.

2 *Framing virtual space*: Therapists should explicitly address how the therapeutic frame translates to the online setting. For example, partners should be encouraged to participate from a private, uninterrupted space to maintain the focus and intimacy of the session.
3 *Engagement strategies*: Online therapy requires creative approaches to sustain engagement. Therapists may incorporate shared digital tools, such as drawing or sketching relational dynamics on virtual whiteboards, to enhance understanding and interaction.
4 *Managing environmental factors*: Couples often join sessions from their shared home environment, which can introduce dynamics that are not present in in-person therapy. For instance, the presence of children or shared living spaces can add layers of complexity to the therapeutic process. Therapists must navigate these dynamics thoughtfully.

Despite its challenges, online psychoanalytic couple therapy offers several unique advantages:

1 *Increased accessibility*: Couples in remote areas or with mobility limitations can access therapy without the need for travel. This can be particularly beneficial for those with demanding schedules or caregiving responsibilities.
2 *Insights into the home environment*: Online therapy provides a window into the couple's living environment, offering additional context for understanding their relational dynamics. Therapists can observe interactions in a more natural setting, which may inform the therapeutic process.
3 *Continuity of care*: The flexibility of online therapy allows for continuity in times of crisis, such as during the COVID-19 pandemic. Partners can maintain therapeutic progress despite external disruptions.
4 *Anonymity and comfort*: For some couples, the physical distance provided by online therapy can reduce feelings of vulnerability, facilitating a willingness to explore difficult emotions and topics. High-conflict couples can avoid the threat of escalating their conflict by connecting from two different rooms.

Online Analytic Groups

Many group therapy schools exist in the group therapy field, ranging from psychoeducational to interpersonal (following Yalom's model) to psychodynamic. I will relate only to psychodynamic and group analytic groups (explained below) when discussing online analytic groups. Psychodynamic therapy groups are a form of group psychotherapy rooted in psychoanalytic theory, where members explore unconscious patterns, emotional conflicts, and relational dynamics within a safe group setting. The group acts as a microcosm of members' external relationships, enabling insight, self-awareness, and personal growth through interactions, transference, and feedback from others and the therapist. The theory and practice of these groups are described in Rutan, Stone, and Shay (2014). They are common in the United States.

Group analysis is "a form of psychotherapy by the group, of the group, including its conductor" (Foulkes 1975, p. 3). It is a psychotherapeutic approach that emphasizes the healing potential of group interactions. It integrates psychoanalytic principles, systems theory, and sociology to explore how individuals function within a group context. The group serves as a dynamic, interactive space where members uncover unconscious processes, relational patterns, and shared experiences. Through dialogue, reflection, and mutual feedback, participants gain deeper self-awareness and interpersonal understanding, fostering psychological growth and transformation. One of the main differences between group analysis and psychodynamic group therapy (or any other group modality) is the emphasis on unconscious social forces that shape the individual members' and the group's behavior (the "Social Unconscious", see Hopper and Weinberg, 2011, 2015, 2017). This group modality is practiced mainly in the United Kingdom, Europe, and Israel.

For those who are acquainted in Yalom's frame of reference that is practiced all around the world, and wonder why it wasn't included in the psychodynamic group modalities, let me explain that Yalom focuses only on the here-and-now and is not interested in the past experiences that shaped the behaviors and unconscious dynamics of the person (he does try to bring behaviors to awareness, but being unaware is not the same as being unconscious). Since the psychoanalytic approach emphasizes the dynamic and past origins of behaviors, I excluded Yalom's theoretical group approach from this book.

An important difference between the outcome determinants in individual and group therapy is that in individual therapy the therapeutic alliance is the factor that is most highly correlated with positive outcomes (Horvath & Symonds, 1991). The main predictor for the group's success is not the relationship between group members and the therapist, but the connection among the group members themselves, namely the group cohesion (Burlingame et al., 2018).

The current body of research on cohesion in online groups is still lacking. The most current review (Andrews et al., 2024) identified 33 articles that included information regarding group therapy online. They concluded that there is a growing but incomplete body of knowledge that informs the group therapist regarding the ethical delivery of groups online. Weinberg (2021) shares his experience that it takes longer for the group to become cohesive, but when it develops, the online group becomes no less effective, intimate, and meaningful than when led in-person.

Researchers have studied the efficacy of online group psychotherapy in different populations, including individuals with depression, anxiety, and post-traumatic stress disorder. A meta-analysis of 17 studies found that online group therapy was effective in reducing symptoms of anxiety, depression, and PTSD (Andersson et al., 2016).

Marmarosh et al. (2023) amended Burlingame et al.'s (2001) six empirically supported principles for group therapists for online therapy groups. Among other suggestions, she reminds us that the therapist needs to be sensitive to the online nature of interventions and can model how to be more personal and connected in online groups. She adds that group therapists may need to be more active at bringing in members who may disengage during the sessions, since it is more challenging to express emotions online, and it is much easier for a member to pull away and withdraw.

Unfortunately, specific research about group analysis online is still missing and is very much needed. Weinberg (2025) brought arguments about why online analytic groups should be considered valid as part of group analytic training. His arguments cover theoretical, practical, research, and experiential perspectives. Friedman (2023) writes that communicational and relational characteristics of group analysis will have to translate from the usual face-to-face group into the online format. He suggests that group-analytic specific concepts need to be transposed in the online format. He goes through the main important group analytic concepts and processes, such as exchange (which is the ability to give and take in interpersonal situations), building a group-analytic matrix, mirroring and resonance, and shows how to apply them online. As for resonance, he writes: "Because of visceral aspects of resonance, its impact online might be somewhat milder than in f2f meetings, but still will be influential" (Friedman, 2023, p. 102).

Below is a group vignette exemplifying some of the challenges of online group analysis and describing how an appropriate analytic approach in dealing with these challenges can lead to meaningful work.[1]

After missing the previous session, Sarah appeared on the screen in the next session, sitting in the back seat of a cab and using her cell phone to connect to the group. The group members expressed their thoughts regarding her absence from the previous session, but nobody mentioned that she was in a car with a driver. The group analyst wondered whether he was the only one noticing that Sarah was in a cab on her phone and asked how people felt about it.

Nora said that she was worried about confidentiality and did not feel safe, to which Sarah replied that it was okay, because she did not know the driver. This comment enraged some group members who felt that Sarah was not being considerate of their privacy. Fiona was concerned that Sarah would not be able to emotionally connect with the group. Hella noted that Sarah did not want to miss this group session again and had made the effort to connect, despite being on the road. Sarah was touched by this empathic response and acknowledged that she wanted to get to an important meeting, but did not want to miss the group session. She asked the group what to do. Nora wanted Sarah to leave the session and come back next time.

David said that Sarah had violated the agreement they had all made when entering the group.

The group analyst suggested that Sarah leave the group session and join the next session. Sarah became angry and shouted that the leader and group were inhumane and that she did not want to participate anymore. She disconnected and disappeared from the screen. Some people expressed anger with Sarah and with the group leader. Others were afraid that they would also be rejected if they deviated from group norms. The group analyst encouraged expression of all feelings, saying that safety is about the freedom to discuss difficult issues in addition to setting boundaries.

At the next meeting, Sarah showed up at home, to everyone's relief. The group analyst suggested discussing the dramatic events from the prior meeting. Sarah thanked everyone for the previous meeting; she had thought a lot about what had happened and about her strong emotional reaction. She said she remembered being rejected by her family and by peers. Other members who had felt rejected throughout their lives empathized with her and shared their rejection memories. These two meetings became a turning point for the group and increased the members' ability to express differences and to feel safe in opening.

Note

1 The case appears in Weinberg (2021).

Chapter 7

Training for Online Psychodynamic Psychotherapy

Introduction

The rise of online psychodynamic psychotherapy marks a significant evolution in mental health treatment, offering unprecedented access and convenience through digital platforms. This modality has expanded rapidly, particularly during global events such as the COVID-19 pandemic, highlighting its potential to overcome geographical and logistical barriers to care. However, the digital environment introduces unique challenges that necessitate specialized training for therapists.

Traditional psychotherapy training typically emphasizes in-person interactions within the controlled setting of a therapist's office. The shift to online therapy introduces complexities related to technology, communication, and the therapeutic relationship. Therapists must adapt their skills and techniques to engage effectively with clients in a virtual space, manage technical issues, and navigate the altered dynamics of online communication. The nuances of nonverbal communication, the importance of establishing a secure and private environment remotely, and the management of technological disruptions all require specific attention in training curricula.

This chapter examines the critical need for comprehensive training in online psychodynamic psychotherapy. It explores the challenges and opportunities presented by the digital environment and emphasizes the importance of developing specific competencies to ensure effective and ethical practice. Key areas of focus

DOI: 10.4324/9781003503514-7

include cultivating flexibility and creativity to foster presence, overcoming the limitations of remote communication, engaging with the virtual body, understanding transference and countertransference dynamics in the online setting, addressing ethical considerations, and mastering technological competencies. By addressing these elements, training programs can equip therapists to deliver high-quality care and navigate the complexities of online practice with confidence and skill. Online individual therapy training programs should prioritize adaptation to the distinct attributes of the virtual environment. Furthermore, this chapter looks at the role of ongoing professional development and the integration of research into training curricula to ensure therapists are well prepared to meet the evolving demands of online practice.

The Need for Training in Online Psychotherapy

Even before the surge in telehealth adoption during the COVID-19 pandemic, research indicated a growing need for specialized training in telehealth practices (Callan et al., 2017). Glueckauf et al. (2018) revealed that approximately 90% of psychologists believed that mental health practitioners should receive training on the clinical, legal, and ethical aspects of telehealth. This consensus highlights the recognition within the field that providing therapy remotely requires a distinct skill set and an understanding of unique considerations.

Research suggests that therapists often experience uncertainty regarding their capabilities in online therapy, which can detrimentally affect their therapeutic presence and efficacy. Many practitioners have reported needing training on technical issues related to delivering online mental health services. The integration of technology into therapy introduces a new layer of complexity, requiring therapists to be proficient in using various platforms, troubleshooting technical difficulties, and ensuring the security and privacy of client data. Self-assessments revealed that around 40% of psychologists felt they lacked sufficient telehealth training, and about half reported inadequate skills in handling emergencies during online sessions. These findings underscore the gap between the demand for online therapy and the availability of adequate training resources for practitioners.

In a pilot study (Messina & Loffler-Stastka, 2021), therapists reported feeling less proficient in certain clinical skills when working online compared to in-person settings. This highlights the importance of tailoring training programs to address the specific challenges that therapists face in the virtual environment. Sampaio et al. (2021) found a substantial increase in telepsychology use during COVID-19 (from 39% to 98%). The conclusion of the researchers was that a number of therapists still had ethical, training, and personal concerns regarding the use of telepsychology, and gaps in therapists' knowledge on these topics were evident, indicating a strong need for increased telepsychology training for therapists in the future.

The online setting differs significantly from the traditional office environment. The therapist has limited control over the patient's environment and cannot directly ensure a holding environment on the patient's side of the screen. Therefore, training programs should emphasize educating patients on creating a safe and private space for online sessions. Instructions should cover how to minimize distractions, maintain privacy, and stay focused during the session. This includes providing guidance on setting up a dedicated therapy space, using headphones to enhance privacy, and ensuring that family members or housemates are aware of the importance of confidentiality during sessions.

The therapist needs to adapt to the technological dimension. Technology influences the therapeutic process, evoking associations and unconscious fantasies that add a technological layer to the interaction. The therapist should be aware of technology's impact and learn to interpret its influence. For example, camera placement can affect perceived eye contact, and technical difficulties can disrupt the therapeutic alliance. Training should include exercises to help therapists become more attuned to these technological nuances and develop strategies for addressing them in therapy.

Harris and Tylim (2018) noted that the concept of the therapeutic framework has evolved due to social, cultural, and technological forces. In online therapy, technology profoundly shapes the setting. Just as attention to the physical environment (lighting, sound, decor) enhances in-person therapy, similar considerations apply online. Addressing technical challenges and exploring the patient's associations and fantasies related to the online setting can help re-create a safe and holding environment. Training programs should incorporate analysis of the setting itself as a key element of psychotherapeutic technique in the digital space. This includes helping therapists understand how digital interfaces, such as video screens and audio quality, can impact the therapeutic relationship and the client's experience.

Key Competencies for Online Psychodynamic Therapists

To practice online psychodynamic psychotherapy effectively, therapists must cultivate a specific set of competencies that address the unique demands of the virtual environment. These competencies can be broadly categorized into the following.

1 Clinical Adaptation

Flexibility: Adapting therapeutic techniques to suit the online setting, including managing unexpected disruptions and technical issues.

Presence: Maintaining a sense of connection and engagement with clients despite the physical distance.

Engagement with the virtual body: Helping clients connect with their physical sensations and experiences in the absence of in-person contact.

Management of transference and countertransference: Recognizing and addressing transference and countertransference dynamics that may be influenced by the technological medium.

2 Ethical Awareness

Confidentiality: Ensuring the privacy and security of client information in the digital environment.

Informed consent: Obtaining informed consent from clients regarding the risks and benefits of online therapy, as well as the use of technology.

Boundary management: Maintaining appropriate professional boundaries in the online setting, including managing social media interactions and electronic communication.

Emergency management: Developing protocols for handling emergencies that may arise during online sessions, such as suicidal ideation or medical crises.

3 Technological Proficiency

Platform familiarity: Becoming proficient in using various online therapy platforms, including videoconferencing software, secure messaging systems, and electronic health records.

Troubleshooting: Developing the ability to troubleshoot common technical issues, such as audio and video problems, connectivity issues, and software glitches.

Data security: Implementing measures to protect client data from unauthorized access, including using strong passwords, encrypting electronic communications, and complying with relevant privacy regulations.

Flexibility

An online group member seemed quite constrained and quiet for a long time in the group sessions. When the group inquired what was happening to him and why he was so quiet and passive, he revealed that he was having serious problems in his marriage, but since he was connecting from home and the walls in his house are thin, he did not feel that it was safe to talk about his intimate issues and difficulties in his relationship with his wife when she was behind the wall. The group therapist (me) suggested that he go to his parked car and connect from there.

Therapists must be flexible to adapt to the unique conditions of online therapy. This requires moving away from rigid, traditional approaches. A therapist should acknowledge that online therapy differs from in-person therapy, with factors such as the setting being less controlled, communication failures being more likely, and establishing a sense of safety potentially being more challenging.

Flexibility involves relaxing the usual rigid boundaries and rules of traditional psychotherapy. The therapist needs to recognize that the patient controls a significant portion of the setting. Sharing responsibility with the patient for creating a safe environment can promote adult coping skills and reduce regression. While this shift can be advantageous or disadvantageous depending on the patient, training programs should explore these dynamics and their potential consequences. Clearly, the online setting is different from the traditional one in our office. In my co-edited book (Weinberg and Rolnick, 2020) and in my writing (Weinberg, 2020a) I related to the fact that the therapist cannot create the conditions on the patient's side of the screen to guarantee a holding environment. Thus, the therapist should educate the patients on how to create a safe environment. This is an important issue that should be emphasized again and again and should become part of the online training: Prepare your patient for the online meeting, and instruct them on how to keep privacy, stay focused, etc.

Incorporating case examples into training can help therapists develop greater flexibility in their approach. For instance, role-playing scenarios where the therapist must navigate unexpected disruptions, such as a pet entering the frame or a sudden loss of internet connection, can help build resilience and adaptability. Additionally, discussing ethical dilemmas specific to online therapy, such as managing confidentiality in a digital environment or handling emergency situations remotely, can enhance a therapist's capacity for flexible problem-solving.

Flexibility also extends to the therapist's mindset. Online therapy may require therapists to be more adaptable in their theoretical approach, integrating different techniques and interventions to meet the unique needs of each client. This might involve combining psychodynamic principles with cognitive-behavioral strategies or mindfulness practices to address specific challenges that arise in the online setting.

Presence

Therapeutic presence involves bringing one's whole self to the engagement with the client, being fully in the moment with and for the client, with little self-centered purpose or goal in mind (Geller & Greenberg, 2012). It requires being deeply rooted in the moment on a physical, emotional, cognitive, relational, and spiritual level. Clients perceive this presence as creating safety, making them feel met and understood (Geller, 2023). Maintaining presence can be more challenging online due to distractions and the screen barrier. However, therapists can learn techniques to enhance their online presence.

1. Use Yourself More

Appropriate self-disclosure can help create presence. Sharing here-and-now feelings toward the patient can be helpful. However, it's important to distinguish between appropriate self-disclosure (feelings in the present moment) and sharing personal history. Training should include guidelines on ethical self-disclosure and emphasize the importance of maintaining appropriate boundaries. This may involve discussing the difference between self-involving and self-revealing disclosures, as well as the potential impact of therapist self-disclosure on the therapeutic relationship.

2. Pay Close Attention to Facial Expressions

Observing the patient's facial expressions (which are often more visible online due to the close-up view) can help identify unexpressed feelings. Taking responsibility for mistakes and empathic failures can also enhance presence. Training can incorporate exercises that focus on recognizing subtle facial cues and interpreting nonverbal communication in the online environment. This may involve using video recordings of therapy sessions to analyze facial expressions and body language, as well as practicing active listening skills to enhance empathic understanding.

3. Use of Imagination

Imagination activates the brain in ways that mimic real experience. Encouraging the patient to use their imagination can increase the experiential component of therapy and enhance the sense of presence. Therapists can be trained to use guided imagery techniques or encourage clients to visualize their internal experiences to deepen their emotional connection and sense of presence. This may involve exploring the use of metaphors, storytelling, and creative expression to facilitate emotional processing and insight.

An example of the use of imagination from an analytic group follows. *A group member expressed irritation and sadness about the loss of sitting in a circle, not sensing the "real" presence of the participants. She complained about the squares that appear on her screen whose positions change every meeting and sometimes even during the meeting (whenever someone's internet disconnects). My response as the group leader was: "Please close your eyes and imagine that we are now sitting in a circle in the same room. Who would you like to sit beside you? Who would you like to sit across the room far away from you?" Using imagination and discussing her fantasy about possible group seating instigated a deep conversation about intimacy, closeness, disconnection, and distance between group members.*

4. Naming Sensations and Observations

Explicitly naming sensations, observations, and people's names can strengthen connections, as subtle cues are often lost online. Encouraging the patient to be specific in their references can reduce ambiguity. Training can include exercises where therapists practice articulating their observations and sensations in the moment, fostering a greater sense of connection with the client. This may involve using mindfulness practices to enhance sensory awareness and developing the ability to describe internal experiences in a clear and evocative manner.

Research (Haddouk, 2015) indicates that psychological presence is crucial for building and maintaining therapeutic alliances online. Training should focus on enhancing therapeutic presence, especially for therapists who feel less competent or experience more difficulties in the online setting. This might involve mindfulness practices, self-reflection exercises, and role-playing scenarios that allow therapists to practice and refine their ability to be fully present with their clients in the virtual space.

Engaging the Virtual Body

One of the major challenges in online therapy stems from the absence of the physical body and its immediacy and the loss of nonverbal communication. The lack of body-to-body communication is a significant loss. The body serves as a gateway to connect with one's full human experience.

Training should address how therapists can help patients stay connected to their bodies even when physically separated. Some potential techniques include:

- *Encouraging movement*: Suggesting patients move or stretch during sessions can help them stay grounded in their bodies.
- *Focusing on breathing*: Guiding patients through breathing exercises can help them regulate their emotions and connect with their physical sensations.
- *Paying attention to posture*: Helping patients become aware of their posture and body language can provide valuable insights into their emotional state.
- *Using sensory awareness*: Encouraging patients to notice and describe their sensory experiences (e.g., what they see, hear, smell, taste, and touch) can help them stay present and connected to their bodies.

In Chapter 3, in the section titled Modifications, Creative Solutions, and Clinical Sensitivity, I suggested more techniques to bring the body online, such as inviting the patient to report their body sensations or using "body-oriented metaphorical language." Therapists who were trained in the somatic experience, sensorimotor (Ogden and Goldstein, 2020), or Gestalt approaches know how to do it well. The passive analytic approach is less suitable for engaging the body in online therapy and the training should help therapists become more active in asking patients to get closer to or further away from the camera, move in the room, etc. All these techniques should be taught and practiced in any training for online therapy. Additionally, training can explore how therapists can use their own bodies to communicate empathy and understanding in the online setting. This might involve paying attention to their facial expressions, posture, and gestures, and using these nonverbal cues to convey warmth, compassion, and attunement. Training programs can include exercises in mirroring and attunement, helping therapists to consciously use their own physical presence to enhance the therapeutic relationship.

Transference and Countertransference

Transference and countertransference dynamics are integral to psychodynamic psychotherapy, and they take on unique dimensions in the online setting. Training should address how therapists can recognize and manage these dynamics effectively in the virtual space.

Transference in Online Therapy

In online therapy, transference may be influenced by the technological medium. For example, a client might project certain qualities onto the therapist based on their online presence, such as their profile picture, website design, or technical proficiency. Additionally, the client's fantasies about the therapist's life outside the session may be heightened due to the lack of physical context. The therapist's technological competence or lack thereof may also become a focus of transference, with clients attributing certain qualities to the therapist based on their perceived digital skills.

Training should help therapists become aware of these potential transference dynamics and explore how they might impact the therapeutic relationship. This might involve discussing case examples where transference issues have emerged in online therapy and practicing techniques for addressing these issues effectively. This can include role-playing exercises that simulate common transference scenarios and provide opportunities for therapists to practice their responses.

Countertransference in Online Therapy

Countertransference, the therapist's emotional reactions to the client, can also be amplified in the online setting. Therapists may experience feelings of isolation, detachment, or anxiety due to the physical distance and the limitations of online communication. Additionally, technical difficulties or disruptions during sessions can trigger frustration or impatience, which may unconsciously influence the therapist's responses to the client. The therapist's own relationship with technology and their comfort level with the online environment can also impact their countertransference reactions.

Training should provide therapists with opportunities to explore their own countertransference reactions in the online setting. This might involve self-reflection exercises, supervision sessions, and peer consultation groups where therapists can share their experiences and receive support and guidance. This should include discussions about the impact of the online environment on the therapist's emotional state and strategies for managing these challenges.

Ethical Considerations

Practicing psychodynamic psychotherapy online introduces a range of ethical considerations that therapists must be prepared to address. Training programs should provide comprehensive coverage of these issues, including the following.

1 *Confidentiality and data security*: Ensuring the privacy and security of client information is paramount in online therapy. Therapists must be knowledgeable about relevant privacy regulations (e.g., HIPAA in the United States, General Data Protection Regulation, GDPR, in Europe) and implement appropriate measures to protect client data from unauthorized access. This includes using secure communication platforms, encrypting electronic communications, and storing client records in a secure manner.

2 *Informed consent*: Obtaining informed consent from clients regarding the risks and benefits of online therapy is essential. Clients should be informed about the limitations of online communication, the potential for technical difficulties, and the steps the therapist will take to protect their privacy and confidentiality. The informed consent process should also address issues such as emergency management and the therapist's scope of practice in the client's location.
3 *Boundary management*: Maintaining appropriate professional boundaries can be more challenging in the online setting. Therapists must be mindful of their online presence and avoid engaging in dual relationships with clients through social media or other electronic platforms. Clear guidelines should be established regarding communication outside of scheduled sessions, as well as the therapist's availability and response time.
4 *Emergency management*: Therapists practicing online must have protocols in place for handling emergencies that may arise during sessions, such as suicidal ideation or medical crises. This includes developing a safety plan with the client, identifying local emergency resources, and ensuring that the therapist is able to respond effectively in a crisis situation.
5 *Scope of practice*: Therapists practicing online must be aware of the legal and regulatory requirements in both their own jurisdiction and the client's location. This includes ensuring that the therapist is licensed to practice in the client's state or country and that they are familiar with the relevant laws and ethical guidelines.

Technological Competencies

In addition to clinical and ethical considerations, therapists practicing online psychodynamic psychotherapy must also possess a certain level of technological competence. Training programs should provide instruction and hands-on experience in the following areas.

1 *Platform familiarity*: Therapists should be proficient in using various online therapy platforms, including videoconferencing

software, secure messaging systems, and electronic health records. Training should include instruction on how to use these platforms effectively, as well as troubleshooting common technical issues.

2 *Troubleshooting*: Therapists should be able to troubleshoot common technical problems that may arise during online sessions, such as audio and video issues, connectivity problems, and software glitches. Training should provide practical tips and strategies for resolving these issues quickly and efficiently.
3 *Data security*: Therapists should be knowledgeable about data security best practices and implement measures to protect client data from unauthorized access. This includes using strong passwords, encrypting electronic communications, and storing client records in a secure manner. Training should also cover the use of firewalls, antivirus software, and other security tools.
4 *Hardware and software*: Therapists should have a basic understanding of the hardware and software requirements for online therapy, including computer equipment, internet connections, and software applications. Training should provide guidance on selecting appropriate equipment and software, as well as optimizing system performance for online sessions.

Recommendations for Structuring Effective Training Programs

To ensure that therapists are adequately prepared for the challenges and opportunities of online psychodynamic psychotherapy, training programs should incorporate the following elements.

1 *Didactic instruction*: This provides therapists with a solid foundation in the theory and practice of online therapy, including ethical and legal considerations, technical aspects, and the unique dynamics of the virtual therapeutic relationship. It should include lectures, readings, and discussions that cover the key concepts and principles of online psychodynamic psychotherapy.

2 *Experiential learning*: This offers opportunities for therapists to practice their skills in a safe and supportive environment, such as role-playing scenarios, simulated online sessions, and peer consultation groups. It should include opportunities for therapists to practice using various online therapy platforms, troubleshooting technical issues, and managing ethical dilemmas.
3 *Supervision*: This provides ongoing supervision from experienced online therapists who can offer guidance, feedback, and support. It should include individual supervision, group supervision, and live observation of online therapy sessions.
4 *Self-reflection*: Therapists should be encouraged to engage in self-reflection exercises to explore their own biases, assumptions, and emotional reactions in the online setting. This should include journaling, mindfulness practices, and other techniques for promoting self-awareness.
5 *Continuing education*: Therapists should be offered continuing education opportunities to help them stay up-to-date with the latest research, best practices, and technological advancements in online therapy. This should include workshops, conferences, and online courses that cover emerging trends and issues in the field.
6 *Personal therapy*: Therapists should be encouraged to engage in their own personal therapy (preferably online, to feel the experience of being in therapy behind the screen) and to explore their own emotional issues and develop greater self-awareness. This is particularly important for therapists practicing psychodynamic psychotherapy, as personal therapy can help them to better understand their own transference and countertransference reactions.

Integrating Research into Training

To ensure that training programs for online psychodynamic psychotherapy are evidence-based and effective, it is essential to integrate research findings into the curriculum. This includes the following.

1 *Staying up-to-date with the literature*: Training programs should incorporate readings and discussions of current research on online therapy, including studies on its effectiveness, ethical implications, and best practices.
2 *Critically evaluating research*: Therapists should be trained to evaluate research findings critically and to assess the strengths and limitations of different studies. This includes understanding research methodologies, statistical analyses, and the potential for bias.
3 *Conducting research*: Training programs should encourage therapists to participate in research on online therapy, either by conducting their own studies or by collaborating with researchers at academic institutions. This can help to advance the field and to develop new and innovative approaches to online practice.
4 *Applying research to practice*: Therapists should be trained to apply research findings to their clinical practice. This includes using evidence-based techniques and interventions, as well as monitoring client outcomes to assess the effectiveness of their work.

Conclusion

Training for online individual psychodynamic psychotherapy requires a comprehensive approach that addresses the unique challenges and opportunities presented by the digital environment. By cultivating flexibility, fostering presence, engaging with the virtual body, understanding transference and countertransference dynamics, addressing ethical considerations, and mastering technological competencies, therapists can effectively adapt their skills and techniques to meet the needs of clients in the online setting. Effective training programs should incorporate didactic instruction, experiential learning, supervision, self-reflection, continuing education, and personal therapy to ensure that therapists are well-equipped to provide high-quality online mental health care. As the field of online therapy continues to evolve, ongoing training and professional development will be essential for therapists to remain competent and ethical in their practice. By integrating research into training curricula, we can ensure that therapists are using evidence-based approaches and that the field continues to advance in a responsible and ethical manner.

Chapter 8

The Future of Online Psychoanalysis

Trends and Predictions

The Current State of Online Psychoanalysis

As described in detail in the previous chapters, online psychoanalysis involves using digital platforms for therapeutic sessions, typically through videoconferencing. It maintains the core principles of psychoanalysis – exploring unconscious processes, transference, and relational dynamics – while adapting to the limitations and opportunities of virtual communication. The advent of the internet and advances in communication technologies have enabled psychoanalysis to transcend geographical boundaries. Initially, online therapy sessions were conducted through emails and chat rooms. However, with the proliferation of high-speed internet and smartphones, videoconferencing became the preferred medium, offering a more personal and effective means of communication.

Despite challenges, such as reduced nonverbal cues and the absence of shared physical space, many practitioners and clients report successful therapeutic outcomes, underscoring the potential of this medium. Platforms like Zoom, Doxy.me, Google Meet, and specialized psychotherapy tools have become staples in online psychoanalysis, offering features such as secure video sessions, session recording (with consent), and asynchronous communication. These technologies have paved the way for a more accessible and flexible approach to psychoanalysis, breaking down barriers related to geography, mobility, and stigma. The COVID-19 pandemic further accelerated the adoption of online psychoanalysis.

DOI: 10.4324/9781003503514-8

With lockdowns and social distancing measures in place, many therapists and clients turned to digital platforms. Studies have shown that online therapy can be as effective as in-person sessions, leading to its increased acceptance and legitimacy within the mental health community.

This chapter explores the current state of online psychoanalysis, its growth, and predictions for its future, focusing on emerging trends such as virtual reality (VR), augmented reality (AR), artificial intelligence-assisted (AI-assisted) therapy, wearable technology integration, remote biofeedback, and automation.

Emerging Trends in Online Psychoanalysis

The rapid growth of telehealth has spurred innovations that promise to revolutionize online psychoanalysis further. Below are key trends and predictions.

1. Immersive Therapy with VR and AR

Virtual reality and augmented reality have the potential to revolutionize and transform the therapeutic landscape by creating and providing immersive environments for psychoanalytic work. VR can create simulated scenarios that allow patients to confront and work through their fears and anxieties in a controlled and safe setting. Therapists can use VR to simulate scenarios that evoke unconscious material, allowing clients to explore memories, fears, and desires in a controlled and safe virtual space. Clients might revisit significant life events or symbolic environments that represent their inner world, guided by the therapist. For instance, exposure therapy for phobias can be conducted in a VR setting where patients face their fears virtually before confronting them in real life.

Augmented reality could project the therapist's image into the client's environment, fostering a greater sense of connection and immediacy. AR can enhance real-world environments with therapeutic prompts and interactive elements, making therapy more engaging and effective. For example, AR can help patients with social anxiety practice interactions in real-world settings enhanced with supportive cues and guidance. Such immersive technologies could bridge some gaps inherent in online therapy, such as the lack of shared physical space, and create new opportunities for experiential and symbolic work.

2. Three-Dimensional Conversation

As mentioned a few times throughout this book, one of the main difficulties in online therapy is the disembodied environment. The body-to-body interaction is missing online. As much as I suggested ways to overcome this shortcoming, online interaction still occurs in two dimensions (2D). Companies around the world are already working on projects to create an online three-dimensional (3D) illusion. These projects aim to revolutionize videoconferencing by making it feel like people are having a face-to-face conversation with someone in 3D, rather than looking at a flat image on a screen. Instead of just a single 2D camera, it uses an array of cameras to capture the therapist's image from multiple angles. AI uses these multiple camera feeds to create a real-time, detailed 3D model of the therapist. It's not just a flat image with some depth effects; it's a volumetric representation that appears to have actual depth and presence.

The goal is to make the remote conversation feel as natural as possible. This includes being able to make eye contact, read subtle nonverbal cues such as gestures and facial expressions, and generally feel a greater sense of "presence" with the other person. This feature is designed to overcome the limitations of traditional 2D video calls by creating a "magic window" that makes it seem like a life-sized, three-dimensional version of the other person is right there in the room with you.

3. Real-Time Translation

This new feature, which has already been announced, is real-time speech translation, allowing participants to speak different languages and still understand each other seamlessly. This feature expands therapy services that psychodynamic psychotherapists can provide to many patients in countries that have been limited so far by the "language barrier." However, before using this feature to reach patients in other countries, therapists should check the legal status of providing psychological services in countries where they are not licensed. This service also might not be compliant with HIPAA regulations as it uses the cloud for translation.

4. AI-Assisted Therapy

The recent AI boom of the 2020s that led to the rapid scaling and public releases of large language models (LLMs) such as ChatGPT stormed public discourse and ignited the imagination of people from scientists to artists, but also raised fears of losing control and of machines taking over the world. Concerns about the potential risks and ethical implications of advanced AI have emerged, prompting debate about the future of AI and its impact on society. Psychoanalysts may also experience an upheaval following the recent increasing use of generative artificial intelligence (GAI).

Below is a related case study.

Several years ago, I received a phone call from another therapist in town who wanted to refer one of her patients to me. I asked her about the details of the case, and she told me that she had been treating him for two years for his PTSD symptoms, and his symptoms improved some, but recently he developed feelings toward her as a maternal figure and that is why she wanted to refer him to me. I was quite surprised about this reason and told her that according to my therapeutic approach, this is a common transference reaction, and this is where therapy starts, not ends. She responded: "I am a CBT therapist. I don't know how to deal with transference. You are well-known in town as a psychodynamic therapist. You will know how to deal with it." Although this was quite a shocking approach, after trying to convince her to continue working with him, I understood that she could not work through her countertransference, and so I agreed to see him once to make up my mind whether I could work with him. He came to this session and stayed in therapy with me for seven years.

It took several years for this patient to overcome his disappointment, hurt, and abandonment feelings toward his previous therapist. As I suspected, in his maternal transference he idealized her as a perfect mother, who was supposed to compensate him for his narcissistic biological mother. During their therapy, he was clinging to any sign of special attention, warmth, and positive attitude from his therapist, and, according to his report, she colluded with his fantasy and provided enough evidence for such an attitude. One example that he brought was that when a colleague in her office was burning scent to which he, the patient, was allergic, she became angry with her colleague and demanded him to avoid doing it when this patient was in therapy. He said that he tried to bring to her attention that she encouraged his fantasy about her as an ideal mother, but that she could not discuss it and instead decided that he should not continue therapy with her. She told him that he had "an attachment disorder" that prevented her from continuing to see him. He felt rejected and betrayed.

Clearly, ending therapy, especially the way in which he perceived it, without elaborating and working through the termination process, was a huge blow for this patient. He grew up with a very critical and sadistic father, who blamed him for everything that went wrong in the world, and with an unstable mother who could not function well and was unable to properly respond to his needs. As an example: After his parents divorced when he was 12 years old, he and his brother had to take care of their sister since their mother was dysfunctional and stayed in bed all day. Although he did acknowledge that his symptoms improved during the previous therapy sessions, the blow of her rejection, and his feeling as if he was to blame for this abandonment, made him regress dramatically. He had suicidal thoughts, became depressed and very obsessive, telling me again and again how this therapist "seduced" him to believe that he was her special patient/child. He told me that when he started therapy with her, she took a course about how to handle trauma in therapy, to know how to treat him better. I increased our weekly sessions to twice a week to help him with his crisis.

As therapy progressed, he was able to express more anger toward his previous therapist. In fact, there was a period when he was considering suing her or filing a complaint against her to the psychology board. I had to work with my countertransference not to become reactive and to avoid protecting a colleague who seemed to have made mistakes. I acknowledged and accepted his pain and hurt, tried to shift the focus to his need of an idealized mother, as a response to the deep deprivation he experienced with his own mother. I pointed out that I made mistakes as well. He argued that when I make mistakes, I am ready to acknowledge and discuss them with him, trying to repair them, and this fact made a huge difference for him. Slowly, his suicidal thoughts subsided, although he did not give up his revenge fantasies.

This guy was a computer expert and a "positive hacker" in his profession: He was helping organizations and big companies to be protected from computer and internet security breaches, and from any cyberattacks. He had the knowledge and skill of bypassing computer protective tools, and one of his fantasies was to enter his previous therapist's computer and use her private information against her. He was even considering invading her husband's computer to check whether he had any secrets that he could use, to ruin their marriage. I must admit that for a while I was frightened about what would happen if I failed him and how my privacy might be exposed. Fortunately, his ethical values prevented him from executing any of these fantasies.

Slowly, his anger toward his previous therapist shifted from the need to take revenge on her to a need to expose all therapists as imposters (but not me, at least not directly). He told me that he was checking many therapists' websites and had found out that they all have serious security problems, so that their patients' information could easily be retrieved. One day, he announced that he had found the perfect way to make all therapists unemployed: ***He was going to develop an AI therapist that would never make mistakes,*** *thus driving all therapists out of business. I assume that it was his way of threatening me indirectly since he could not directly attack me, projecting some of his father's dangerous character onto me. After thinking of an appropriate response, I told him: Perhaps I am making a mistake by helping you create a better AI therapist and by this way chasing me and my colleagues out of business, but I want to suggest that in the algorithm of this AI therapist, you insert the option of making mistakes from time to time, but also of knowing how to repair and correct them, instead of creating a program that never makes mistakes. This would be a much more efficient and successful AI therapist.*

I am not going to tell you about the rest of the therapy story (which was quite successful) since the focus of this discussion is the potential use of AI to assist psychoanalytic therapy or even to replace the analyst. This long case study is an introduction to exploring this topic more deeply. As you might have guessed, I believe that even if using AI as a therapist brings positive outcomes, an important human feature will always be missing: Ruptures, mistakes, and repairing them, generating powerful therapeutic processes (and that makes all the difference).

Artificial intelligence is poised to play a significant role in the future of online psychoanalysis. It is already being integrated into psychotherapy through chatbots and automated assessment tools. In online psychoanalysis, AI could play a supportive role, assisting both therapists and clients in the following ways.

- *Session analysis*: AI could analyze session transcripts to identify recurring themes and patterns, emotional tones, and potential unconscious conflicts, providing therapists with insights to guide their interventions.
- *Personalized interventions*: Machine-learning algorithms could suggest tailored interventions based on the client's patterns of speech, emotional expression and needs, and progress over time.
- *Support and accessibility*: AI-powered chatbots and virtual assistants could provide immediate support and resources to patients, making therapy more accessible. AI-powered chatbots could offer supplemental support between sessions, helping clients process emotions or manage crises while maintaining the psychoanalytic frame.

AI can also assist therapists by automating administrative tasks, providing insights into patient progress, improving interventions, and aiding in training new clinicians. This allows therapists to focus more on the therapeutic process and less on routine tasks. In psychological practice, AI chatbots can make therapy more accessible and less expensive. On the research side, artificial intelligence offers new ways to understand human intelligence, while machine learning allows researchers to glean insights from massive quantities of data. While AI will not replace the human therapist, it can enhance the depth and efficiency of psychoanalytic work, particularly in data analysis and continuity of care.

Several articles have been published already exploring the relationship between psychotherapy, psychoanalysis, and using AI, although I have not found research about using AI in psychoanalysis. The number of articles increased recently (asking ChatGPT to find articles about this topic at the beginning of 2025, it found four articles relating to this topic from 2024 to 2025), pointing to the increased interest of psychotherapists in AI. In a systematic review of the literature about the use of AI in the field of mental health, Dehbozorgi et al. (2025) explore the diverse applications of AI in mental health care, highlighting both its benefits and challenges. They conclude that AI-driven tools such as chatbots and predictive modeling have shown promise in improving patient engagement and early detection of mental health conditions. However, ethical considerations such as data privacy and algorithm transparency remain critical challenges. In another review, Avula & Amalakanti (2025) examined the role and potential of AI in psychiatry, highlighting its advantages and challenges. Their conclusion is that AI applications in psychiatry include real-time assessments, speech analysis, and behavioral algorithms for early diagnosis and treatment planning. However, issues such as biased training data and lack of universal validation standards pose significant hurdles.

Haber et al. (2024) examine the significant shift in mental health and psychotherapy with the advent of generative AI capable of processing and generating human-like language, conceptualizing this development as the "fourth narcissistic blow" on humanity. They follow Freud who identified three narcissistic blows inflicted on humanity by science, which pushed humans to confront and abandon long-held naive beliefs of their narcissistic centrality and control over the world. The first blow was the "cosmological" one that followed Copernicus's discovery that Earth is not in the center of the world since it orbits the sun and not the other way around. Darwin's "biological" revelation on evolution presented another blow since humans are related to apes and are just another evolutionary link and not a divine culmination. Freud himself introduced the "psychological" blow, the third blow, with his psychoanalytic theory, suggesting that human beings are not rational thinkers since beneath our perceived rationality lie unconscious drives and conflicts. Following Freud's theory, Haber et al. (2024) discuss AI's potential impact on human self-perception, social relationships, and the therapeutic process. They claim that we are witnessing the emergence of a distinctive triangular dynamic: Therapist, patient, and the AI "third" entity. The new quality AI brings fundamentally changes the balance of the therapeutic relationship.

"The Third" in psychoanalytic literature refers to an emergent space or dynamic that arises between two individuals, often in the therapeutic relationship. It represents something beyond the sum of the analyst's and patient's separate subjectivities, forming an intersubjective or unconscious field that shapes their interactions. Ogden (2004) describes it as a co-created unconscious structure that mediates the therapist-patient relationship, influencing both participants outside their awareness. Benjamin (2004) frames it in relational terms, emphasizing mutual recognition and the shared space that allows for transformation beyond dominance and submission. According to Haber et al. (2024), for the first time, this "third" element becomes tangible, transitioning from a mere conceptual presence to an interactive entity that both therapist and patient can have a dialogue with and not just about. They propose conceptualizing the presence of AI in psychotherapy (and mental health in general) as an artificial third. The artificial third refers to the concrete and symbolic expression of AI in the cultural-political-digital space and its shaping presence in the therapeutic encounter, society, and the self. While the artificial third can appear in therapy as a "transitional space," thus creating a playful space following Winnicott's perception (1953), its influence does not end there: It also shapes our perception of ourselves and the world.

Singh (2024) introduces a framework that views AI systems as comprising three interacting forces: Human desire for identification, logical structures, and machinery. Drawing on Lacanian psychoanalytic theory, he argues that AI represents a new register of identification, extending traditional psychoanalytic concepts such as the mirror stage and Oedipus complex. The paper emphasizes the necessity of integrating human and social sciences to fully comprehend AI behavior. In an interesting switch, looking at the relationship between AI and psychoanalysis from the opposite direction, Possati (2020) posits that psychoanalytic concepts and methods can be instrumental in studying AI and human-AI interactions. He suggests that understanding the "algorithmic unconscious" – the underlying, often opaque processes of AI systems – can benefit from psychoanalytic insights, particularly in interpreting AI behaviors and decision-making processes. The idea of the "algorithmic unconscious" echoes with the "internet unconscious" concept, part of the social unconscious, as mentioned and discussed in length in Chapter 3.

Despite AI's potential, there is still cause for concern. AI tools used in health care have discriminated against people based on their race and disability status. In addition, rogue chatbots have already spread misinformation. These challenges make psychoanalysts cautious in using AI in their work.

5. Wearable Technology

Wearable technology, such as smartwatches and fitness trackers, can provide real-time data on a patient's physical and emotional states. These devices can monitor heart rate, sleep patterns, skin conductance, brain function, and activity levels, offering valuable insights into the patient's well-being. This data can be integrated into therapy sessions, enabling therapists to tailor their approach based on the patient's current condition. For example, a patient's increased heart rate detected during a session might indicate anxiety, prompting the therapist to address it immediately. Over time, the collected data can help track the patient's progress and adjust treatment plans accordingly.

Wearable devices that track physiological data could be integrated into online psychoanalysis to provide real-time biofeedback. This data could inform therapy: Physiological markers of stress or relaxation could help therapists understand clients' unconscious reactions during sessions. The data can also enhance self-awareness: Clients could use wearable devices to track emotional states outside of sessions, fostering greater insight into their patterns of affect and behavior. For example, neurofeedback devices, such as EEG headsets, could be used to explore the mind-body connection in psychoanalysis, offering a new dimension to understanding and processing unconscious material.

6. Remote Biofeedback

Biofeedback is a technique that helps patients gain awareness and control over physiological functions. With advancements in telehealth, biofeedback can be conducted remotely using specialized devices that monitor physiological signals such as brain waves, muscle tension, and skin temperature. Remote biofeedback can be particularly beneficial for patients dealing with stress, anxiety, and chronic pain. By learning to control their physiological responses, patients can improve their mental health and overall well-being. The integration of biofeedback into online psychoanalysis offers a holistic approach to therapy, addressing both mental and physical aspects of health.

7. Automation and Efficiency

Automation in online psychoanalysis can streamline various aspects of therapy, from appointment scheduling to session reminders. Automated systems can handle routine administrative tasks, allowing therapists to focus more on patient care. Additionally, automation can facilitate the delivery of therapeutic content, such as exercises and educational materials, making therapy more efficient and accessible.

Potential applications include:

1. *Scheduling and billing*: Automated systems could seamlessly manage appointments, reminders, and payments.
2. *Session summaries*: AI-powered tools could generate summaries of key themes and insights discussed in sessions, aiding both therapists and clients in tracking progress.
3. *Psychoanalytic training*: Automated simulations and virtual supervision could enhance the training of psychoanalysts by providing realistic case scenarios and instant feedback.

Predictions for the Future

The continued evolution of telehealth will likely result in a more integrated and immersive approach to online psychoanalysis. Below are key predictions:

1 *Hybrid models*: Many therapists may adopt a hybrid model, combining in-person and virtual sessions to balance the benefits of both formats. VR and AR technologies could further enhance these hybrid models.
2 *Global access*: Online psychoanalysis will continue to break down geographical barriers, enabling clients to access specialists worldwide. This will necessitate advancements in cross-cultural competency and multilingual AI tools.
3 *Ethical and legal considerations*: As technology becomes more integrated into psychoanalysis, ethical and legal challenges will arise, particularly around data security, confidentiality, and the therapist-client relationship.
4 *Normalization of technology*: As immersive technologies and AI become commonplace, clients and therapists will grow more comfortable using them, paving the way for deeper and more creative therapeutic work.

Conclusion

The future of online psychoanalysis is promising and rich with possibilities, with advancements in technology paving the way for more immersive, personalized, and effective therapy. As technology continues to evolve, it will expand the boundaries of psychoanalytic practice, offering new tools for exploring the unconscious and fostering therapeutic change. While challenges remain, such as ethical concerns and the need for rigorous training, the integration of VR and AR, AI-assisted tools, wearable technology, remote biofeedback, and automation will transform the landscape of mental health care. As these technologies continue to evolve, they will provide new opportunities for therapists and patients, making psychoanalysis more accessible and impactful than ever before. By embracing these innovations thoughtfully, psychoanalysts can continue to provide meaningful and transformative care in an increasingly digital world.

Most predictions indicate that, within a decade, AI entities will surpass human skills in many areas, leaving billions in the shadow of smarter, more educated, and more talented synthetic beings. Beyond the achievements that artificial intelligence may bring with it in science, medicine, and other fields, what distinguishes it from other technological developments in history is the dizzying acceleration with which it is moving.

The speed at which change is about to occur is out of step with the ability of the economy to adapt to it and with the psychological ability of humans to respond and acclimatize to it. This explains the dystopian fears of mass unemployment, the undermining of educational and vocational training institutions, a radical change in the global economy, a fundamental change in lifestyles and time management, and a re-examination of human-human, human-machine, and truth-seeking relationships. Visions of replacing human psychologists and psychiatrists with AI avatars are constantly gaining fans, and all this alongside a silent anxiety that almost no one dares to voice. It seems that the AI storm is giving rise to a plethora of high-tech and biotech companies that rely on large financial investments and are rushing to join the race to develop technologies that will help identify mental distress, and treat mental disorders, trauma, and loneliness, while accelerating the development of drugs to treat mental disorders.

Artificial intelligence may be characterized by the ability to integrate vast databases – clinical, imaging, laboratory, genetic, speech, voice data, and more – and discern subtleties that humans are unable to discern, thus predicting responses to specific treatments. Psychiatry and psychology, perhaps in the throes of their own future shock, seem to be trying to use artificial intelligence applications to treat yesterday's disorders, without seeming to understand or be sensitive to the fact that this very technology and the momentum with which it is bursting into the world will bring with it new mental and social morbidity whose scope no one is imagining or preparing for.

Chapter 9

Conclusion

Introduction

This book has explored the evolution of psychodynamic psychotherapy within the digital realm, a transformation brought into sharp focus by the COVID-19 pandemic, but whose roots pre-date the global crisis. Initially regarded with skepticism, online psychodynamic work has now gained substantial legitimacy, supported by empirical research, clinical experience, and theoretical innovation. As therapists adapted to unprecedented constraints, many discovered that fundamental psychoanalytic processes, transference, resistance, and unconscious communication, continued to emerge, albeit in reconfigured forms.

The goal of this concluding chapter is to consolidate the insights presented throughout the book, while also addressing some of the more pressing ethical, practical, and philosophical challenges that remain unresolved. It aims to offer a framework for responsible, reflective, and innovative engagement with online psychodynamic therapy, both as a current practice and as a growing area of theoretical and empirical exploration.

The movement of psychoanalysis into the digital space has redefined what it means to "be present," to "hold the frame," and to "listen." This shift has provoked resistance from some quarters, rooted in fears of disembodiment, technological mediation, and loss of traditional containment, but it has also inspired a re-examination of core psychoanalytic principles. As we enter a post-pandemic world in which hybrid and remote work are increasingly

DOI: 10.4324/9781003503514-9

normalized, the relevance of online psychodynamic therapy is only likely to grow.

This transformation is not only technological but also psychological and cultural. Therapists and patients alike have had to renegotiate the nature of intimacy, trust, and the shared symbolic space that underpins analytic work. Online settings present both loss and gain. While the absence of bodily cues may diminish certain communication channels, the digital medium also introduces new metaphoric possibilities, such as the screen as a projective surface and the latency of communication as symbolic delay. The screen becomes a dynamic transitional space, simultaneously distancing and connecting, inviting projections not only onto the analyst but onto the medium itself. Latency, glitches, and visual fragmentation may evoke unconscious processes such as repression, interruption, or dissociation, offering novel avenues for interpretation. The act of "logging in" may symbolically echo entry into a psychic container, while disconnection may mirror rupture or resistance. These metaphors are not merely poetic, they inform how therapists conceptualize transference, containment, and the analytic third in the digital setting, urging a reimagining of foundational concepts in light of technological mediation.

Additionally, the transition to digital platforms has demanded significant self-reflection from therapists about their own embodiment, authority, and presence. The challenge of sustaining psychoanalytic depth across a screen has rekindled interest in some fundamental questions: What is interpretation? What constitutes presence? How do we manage rupture and repair in a context where silence can mean disengagement, disconnection, or emotional withdrawal?

This chapter builds upon those questions to offer a grounded, yet expansive view of how online psychodynamic psychotherapy is reshaping the field, both practically and conceptually.

Summary of Key Points

Throughout this book, a comprehensive picture of the current landscape of online psychodynamic psychotherapy has emerged. The chapters trace both the clinical and theoretical shifts that have occurred as therapists moved their work onto digital platforms. What was once considered an emergency substitute has, in many cases, become a sustained modality of practice. The key themes that have emerged across its chapters include the following.

1. Transformation of the Analytic Setting

The book explores how the psychoanalytic setting has been radically altered by the shift online, challenging traditional assumptions about space, embodiment, and the holding environment. It investigates how the therapeutic frame must be redefined when the office is replaced by the screen.

2. Resistance to Online Work

A central thread is the conscious and unconscious resistance within the psychoanalytic community to accepting online practice. This includes fears of disembodiment, diminished analytic depth, and loss of the "real" encounter, resistances that mirror those seen in patients adapting to virtual spaces.

3. Redefinition of Presence and Absence

The book explores how therapeutic presence can still be cultivated online, though it is shaped differently, through voice, gaze, rhythm, and the reliability of the connection. The book also reflects on the new psychological meanings of absence (e.g., frozen screens, dropped calls) in this disembodied frame.

4. Adaptation of Core Psychoanalytic Concepts

Concepts such as transference, countertransference, resistance, and enactment are shown to persist online, albeit in modified forms. The book emphasizes that symbolic processes continue, and that the digital medium offers new routes for unconscious communication and projection.

5. Embodiment and the Body Ego

Several chapters wrestle with the implications of the absent body in online analysis. The tension between body ego, visual cues, and somatic resonance emerges as a complex area, one where analytic presence must be reconceptualized without physical co-location.

6. Ethical and Practical Challenges

The book addresses the evolving ethical landscape, including confidentiality, technical competence, therapist fatigue, boundary negotiation, and digital equity. It argues for a more explicit and reflective approach to frame-setting in online work.

7. Clinical Creativity and Innovation

Far from seeing online therapy as a diluted form, the book shows how online therapy has pushed therapists to innovate, using metaphor, background, shared rituals, and digital affordances to co-create meaning. This theme challenges the notion that online work is inherently inferior to in-person practice.

8. Re-imagining the Analytic Tradition

Overall, the book invites a reflective engagement with psychoanalysis itself, its traditions, institutions, and assumptions. Rather than rejecting the digital turn, I urge the everyone in this field to integrate it with critical thought, ethical awareness, and clinical depth.

A central insight is the redefinition of the therapeutic frame in online practice. In traditional psychoanalysis, the frame includes physical space, time boundaries, and the embodied co-presence of therapist and patient. Online therapy demands an alternative kind of frame, often co-constructed by therapists and patients. The lack of shared physical space and bodily cues necessitates a more explicit negotiation of boundaries, expectations, and responsibilities. Therapists are required to cultivate "digital presence," a capacity to sustain emotional attunement, containment, and symbolic function despite the absence of corporeal co-regulation. This involves being mindful of tone, rhythm, gaze, and responsiveness across technological mediation. In this context, the frame becomes less about maintaining spatial consistency and more about safeguarding the relational container through clarity, reliability, and mutual reflection.

Another prominent theme is the persistence and transformation of transference and countertransference in online environments. Despite the absence of physical proximity, patients continue to form strong transferential relationships with their therapists. In fact, the screen and the disembodied setting often serve as potent sites of projection. Some patients feel liberated by the physical distance, allowing for a freer flow of associations, while others experience the absence of the body as abandonment or intrusion, depending on their unconscious fantasies. For these individuals, the lack of embodied cues can revive early anxieties about being unseen or unmet. Countertransference too takes on new textures, as therapists grapple with a heightened dependence on facial cues and voice, and with managing their own responses to the "always-on" gaze of the camera. These altered dynamics demand a heightened sensitivity to subtle shifts in affect and rhythm, and a willingness to interpret new symbolic forms of connection and withdrawal. Rather than negating transference and countertransference, the online frame reveals their elasticity and resilience across formats.

The book also highlights how resistance manifests differently online. In a virtual context, patients may more easily disengage, turn off their camera, or avoid discomfort by citing technical issues. Similarly, therapists may unconsciously collude in these avoidant dynamics. These new forms of resistance demand new interpretive and holding capacities on the part of the therapist. As such, online psychotherapy challenges practitioners to refine their attunement in a context where traditional bodily cues and embodied markers of affect, such as shifts in posture, breathing, or subtle gestures, are often diminished or lost altogether. Therapists must rely more heavily on vocal tone, facial expressions, pauses, and digital rhythms to detect avoidance and enactment. Moreover, the medium itself can become part of the resistance: The screen may be idealized, distrusted, or manipulated as an object within the transference. Recognizing these dynamics requires clinicians to develop a nuanced understanding of how psychic defenses adapt and migrate into virtual space, and how therapeutic containment can still be maintained in the face of such challenges.

Finally, the book emphasizes the importance of creativity and flexibility in online practice. Far from being a mere compromise, many therapists have developed innovative ways to use the digital medium to support clinical work. Some have introduced collaborative documents, symbolic artifacts, or the use of the patient's environment in meaning-making. This creative adaptation echoes Freud's own insistence on the need for psychoanalysis to evolve in response to new cultural and technological realities.

The chapters also addressed how concepts such as enactment and projective identification continue to operate robustly online. Patients may experience the therapist's image on screen as an omnipresent observer, or, conversely, as a diminished figure vulnerable to being switched off or minimized. Such dynamics offer new insights into how control, autonomy, and fantasy manifest digitally. Therapists have reported unique forms of enactment tied to digital disruptions, such as patients "disappearing" mid-session as an expression of withdrawal or protest or using connection instability as a way to resist confronting painful material. In some cases, the therapist's own frustration with technology may mirror the patient's emotional volatility, amplifying mutual enactments. These phenomena call for an expanded interpretive repertoire, one that includes the screen, interface, and virtual space as meaningful extensions of the analytic field.

Likewise, group analytic online settings, which previously seemed unimaginable, have emerged as viable and even transformative spaces. In online groups, the matrix of interaction develops differently but is not necessarily weaker. Participants often report deep emotional resonance and relational complexity, supported by the distributed intimacy that the screen affords. However, group leaders must adapt their interventions to work with interruptions, time lags, and the limited visibility of body language. Managing silences, turn-taking, and subgroup formations becomes more deliberate and attuned to the constraints of the medium.

Additionally, phenomena, such as "zoom fatigue," screen-based disengagement, or differential access to technology, introduce new layers to the social unconscious of the group. Yet, despite these challenges, online groups can foster profound experiences of mirroring, resonance, and shared meaning, testament to the resilience of the group process in even the most disembodied settings.

In all cases, therapists have found themselves experimenting, adapting, and deepening their clinical intuition. This spirit of inquiry and clinical creativity is arguably one of the most promising outcomes of the turn to digital therapy, as it allows the analytic frame to be explored rather than merely preserved.

Ethical and Practical Recommendations

The ethical demands of online psychodynamic psychotherapy are complex and evolving. One of the most fundamental shifts required is in the training and supervision of therapists. While traditional psychoanalytic training has emphasized in-person work and physical co-presence, online therapy requires therapists to be explicitly trained in digital ethics, telepresence, and the dynamics of screen-mediated communication. Institutes should include modules on secure communication, privacy standards, and the psychodynamics of technology use, as well as supervision models that account for the nuances of working online. Ethical competence now includes not just the ability to manage transference and maintain boundaries, but also the capacity to navigate digital disruptions with transparency and emotional integrity. Supervision itself may need to be rethought, as both candidates and supervisors may be working in different virtual environments, further complicating the triangulation of analytic learning.

An essential ethical principle in online therapy is the co-construction of the analytic frame. Therapists must work collaboratively with patients to establish the conditions of safety, boundaries, and contingency planning for technical disruptions. This includes agreements about session settings, use of video or audio, handling of disconnections, and protocols for emergencies. Patients should be educated about the limits and possibilities of the online setting, especially in cases of high affect or trauma, where regulation may be more difficult to co-create at a distance. Transparency in these discussions fosters trust and strengthens the therapeutic alliance. Moreover, co-constructing the frame allows for ongoing adjustments as the work deepens, reinforcing a shared sense of responsibility for maintaining the analytic container across shifting technological and emotional landscapes.

Confidentiality and data protection are crucial ethical concerns in online therapy. Therapists must use encrypted platforms, avoid public or insecure networks, and ensure that both they and their patients are in private settings during sessions. Therapists must also consider issues of cultural competence, as online therapy often allows for cross-border work. Awareness of cultural, linguistic, and legal differences is essential for ensuring that therapy remains ethically and clinically sound.

The book also emphasizes the ethical dimensions of transference and boundary management in online spaces. Therapists must be alert to new forms of enactment and dependency that can arise in virtual settings. For instance, the therapist's visible facial expressions during video calls can have a powerful impact, functioning either as reassurance or as intrusion. The absence of physical cues can also heighten the patient's tendency to idealize or devalue the therapist based on minimal stimuli.

In sum, ethical practice in online therapy demands not only technical competence but also enhanced reflexivity, sensitivity to cultural and power dynamics, and the capacity to navigate complex relational processes in a medium that is still evolving.

An additional ethical dimension involves managing the boundary between personal and professional space. Unlike office-based work, online sessions often reveal glimpses of the therapist's or patient's domestic environments. While this can foster intimacy, it can also blur boundaries. Therapists must decide what aspects of their space are visible, what background is appropriate, and how to respond when personal disclosures are made by accident (e.g., a family member entering the room). These micro-events, though seemingly incidental, can carry significant symbolic meaning and activate transferential dynamics. A therapist's visible bookshelf, artwork, or even lighting may become a focus of projection, curiosity, or fantasy. Likewise, intrusions may echo early experiences of invasion, chaos, or lack of containment. Navigating these moments requires ethical tact, interpretive sensitivity, and a willingness to explore their psychic resonance, rather than dismiss them as mere technical mishaps. The therapist's ability to maintain a consistent and thoughtful presence – even in a home setting – becomes part of the ethical holding function of the frame.

Further, therapists must be conscious of the implicit hierarchies and privileges embedded in access to technology. Patients from under-resourced regions may lack access to high-speed internet, quiet environments, or secure devices. The very modality of online therapy risks reinforcing systemic inequalities if practitioners are not proactive in adapting their expectations and practices. Ethical reflection, in this context, includes a commitment to accessibility, flexibility, and social justice.

Therapists also need support systems for managing the psychological toll of sustained online presence. Fatigue, dissociation, and a sense of disconnection are commonly reported among clinicians working exclusively online. Peer support, supervision, and the cultivation of reflective space are vital. Ethics here also include care for the therapist's own capacity to remain attuned, grounded, and emotionally available in digital environments.

Controversies and Ongoing Debates

Online psychodynamic psychotherapy has provoked significant debate within the psychoanalytic community. One of the most contentious issues concerns the role of embodiment. Critics argue that without shared physical space, the therapeutic process loses access to subtle bodily communications, such as posture, breath, micro-expressions, and energetic attunement. These aspects are believed to be central to the experience of intersubjectivity and the development of trust and depth in the analytic relationship.

Another common concern is the erosion of the analytic frame. Detractors suggest that the shift online weakens the holding environment, making it easier for patients to avoid difficult material or for the therapeutic container to be breached by intrusions from home or work life. The screen, rather than serving as a neutral frame, becomes a medium of distortion or overexposure.

Moreover, in remote work, the analyst may be perceived as more accessible or casual, altering the transference dynamic.

The use of technology in therapy also raises fears about the commodification of the therapeutic relationship. Platforms, algorithms, and commercial pressures may subtly shape the therapeutic process in ways that compromise its depth and ethics. Therapists may unconsciously adapt their interventions to fit the expectations of digital efficiency or consumer satisfaction. The danger is that psychoanalysis becomes just another online service, rather than a space for deep psychic transformation.

However, other voices in the field argue that these critiques overlook the adaptability of psychoanalytic thinking. Rather than abandoning foundational concepts, online therapy invites us to reframe them. The screen becomes a new kind of transitional space; the absence of the body heightens the significance of voice, rhythm, and timing. Online therapy does not negate transference or the unconscious, it simply invites us to listen differently, interpret differently, and construct presence in new ways.

The book calls for ongoing empirical research, theoretical innovation, and open dialogue within the psychoanalytic community. It suggests that the future of psychoanalysis depends not on rejecting new modalities but on integrating them thoughtfully, with full awareness of their affordances and limitations.

Another point of contention involves the integrity of the therapeutic relationship itself when mediated by technology. Detractors argue that screens interpose a barrier, flattening affect and diminishing spontaneity. While some of these concerns reflect genuine phenomenological shifts, others may mask an ideological resistance to change, anchored in an idealized image of the consulting room. For example, the sacredness attributed to the couch, the silence, and the subtle embodied cues may reflect not only technical concerns but also unconscious investments in a particular model of authority, ritual, and hierarchy. These investments can sometimes hinder necessary adaptations, as the very elements seen as essential may also exclude or alienate those unable to access traditional settings. By clinging to an ideal of presence rooted solely in the body, the field risks reifying a model of psychoanalysis that may no longer serve an increasingly diverse and digitized world.

The question of training also provokes disagreement. Can analytic candidates truly be trained to conduct deep work online? Is it possible to assess presence, containment, and analytic skill when one's supervisory gaze is also mediated by screens? These questions raise larger concerns about the transmission of the analytic tradition and the role of institutions. Some argue that purely online training dilutes the immersive, intersubjective learning that in-person encounters uniquely afford. Others counter that online training – if thoughtfully designed – can cultivate precisely the kind of reflexivity and adaptability needed for contemporary practice. It allows trainees to develop competencies in digital ethics, telepresence, and flexible framing, while still grappling with core psychoanalytic processes. Rather than replacing embodied experience, online training may serve as a supplement or hybrid pathway that acknowledges the changing conditions of therapeutic work without abandoning the rigor of analytic formation. Institutions are thus challenged to evolve, not by lowering standards, but by broadening what analytic competence can look like in the 21st century.

The debate about online work has also sparked anxieties over professional identity. Is a therapist working from their kitchen table as legitimate as one working from a consulting room steeped in psychoanalytic history? What is lost, and what might be gained, when the mystique of the setting is stripped away? These questions are not simply practical; they cut to the core of psychoanalytic ontology.

Still others worry about depersonalization and burnout. The flatness of screen interactions, the fatigue from sustained digital presence, and the absence of shared silence all take a toll on the clinician. Therapists report a sense of "draining presence," where holding the space online requires greater emotional labor, especially in the absence of traditional cues and somatic co-regulation. These challenges must be acknowledged and addressed if online practice is to be sustainable and humane.

Thus, the controversy is not just about whether online therapy "works," empirical data increasingly confirms that it can, but about what kind of psychoanalysis we want to preserve, and for whom. The conversation is ongoing, and its resolution will likely involve reconfiguration rather than a binary choice.

Future Directions

Looking ahead, the landscape of online psychodynamic psychotherapy is likely to continue evolving in response to cultural, technological, and theoretical developments. The integration of artificial intelligence, virtual reality, and other immersive technologies is already beginning to shape experimental therapeutic environments. These tools may offer new forms of engagement, narrative, and embodiment, particularly for younger or neurodivergent populations. However, they also raise ethical questions about data privacy, algorithmic bias, and the potential automation of aspects of the therapeutic relationship. Can empathy be simulated? Will therapists one day work alongside AI co-facilitators or within virtual environments that replicate analytic settings? While these developments may expand access and creative possibilities, they also challenge the field to articulate its humanistic foundations and safeguard the relational core of psychoanalysis in the face of rapid digital innovation.

Another promising direction is the decolonization of psychoanalytic practice through online platforms. By breaking geographic and institutional barriers, digital therapy creates the possibility of more inclusive, culturally responsive practices. Therapists and patients from diverse backgrounds can engage across borders, enriching the analytic encounter with multiple languages, histories, and symbolic systems. This globalized context challenges the Eurocentric foundations of psychoanalysis and opens space for Indigenous, diasporic, and postcolonial frameworks to enter the analytic conversation. Online platforms can facilitate not only clinical encounters but also training, supervision, and peer exchange across global South and North contexts. However, this expansion must be met with ethical humility and critical reflexivity, recognizing power imbalances, linguistic privilege, and the potential for epistemic colonization even within virtual spaces. True decolonization involves more than access: It requires a willingness to unsettle assumptions and co-create knowledge with those historically excluded from analytic discourse.

Online therapy may also foster new models of group work, supervision, and professional collaboration. The digital space allows for spontaneous, international peer networks, collective training models, and democratized access to psychoanalytic thinking. Online conferences and case discussions enable the circulation of ideas across continents, renewing the intellectual vitality of the field.

The future will likely see a hybridization of modalities, where in-person and online elements are combined in flexible ways. Some analysts may offer blended formats, alternating between physical and virtual sessions. Others may develop entirely new methods of analytic engagement suited to digital natives. In all cases, the emphasis must remain on ethical integrity, clinical depth, and the preservation of psychoanalysis as a space for deep psychic work.

What is needed going forward is a shared commitment to reflective practice, research, and dialogue. Rather than viewing online therapy as a temporary compromise, the field must embrace it as a long-term opportunity for growth, expansion, and innovation.

One promising area for future development lies in online group analytic therapy. While early assumptions held that the analytic matrix required physical co-presence, recent work has demonstrated the viability and, in some cases, the depth of virtual group process. These formats require leaders to adapt their stance: Attending to digital rhythm, moderating speaking turns more actively, and making space for silences without visual cues. Yet the relational field emerges nonetheless, as does the group's capacity to reflect the social unconscious, contain projections, and facilitate meaningful change. Members often report heightened emotional intimacy due to the paradoxical safety of distance, while leaders note increased attunement to vocal tone and narrative structure in the absence of full-body presence. The online setting may also reduce social anxieties for some participants, enabling freer speech and deeper sharing. With continued reflection and empirical study, online group analysis may evolve into a distinct and powerful modality, carrying forward the foundational principles of Foulkesian thinking into a new technological era.

The concept of "telepresence" will also benefit from deeper theoretical elaboration. How do patients experience the therapist's gaze, posture, and attention when mediated by a screen? What unconscious fantasies are activated by latency, glitches, or frozen images? Some theorists have suggested that digital therapy activates a "technological transference," a set of projections onto the medium itself, including fears of surveillance, abandonment, omnipotence, or disembodiment. These novel forms of transference can shape the therapeutic process in ways that are both subtle and profound. A therapist's momentary absence due to a lost connection, for instance, may re-enact early attachment ruptures or narcissistic injuries. Conversely, the perceived immediacy of eye contact via the screen may elicit idealization or overexposure. Understanding these dynamics requires new language and models – ones that consider the interface not merely as a barrier, but as an active participant in the analytic field. As we explore these mediated dimensions of presence, psychoanalysis has the opportunity to develop a richer account of what it means to be seen, heard, and held in a digital world.

Another area of interest lies in integrating trauma-informed perspectives into online psychoanalysis. For patients with complex PTSD, dissociation, or attachment trauma, the disembodied setting may serve as both a protection and a trigger. On the one hand, some patients feel safer in their own space, more empowered to regulate contact and exit when overwhelmed. On the other hand, others may find the lack of physical grounding destabilizing. The therapist's ability to modulate their voice, to create safety through rhythm, predictability, and containment, becomes especially vital. Additionally, the therapist must be sensitive to how the screen may both reflect and distort traumatic transferences – mirroring the distance, fragmentation, or invisibility of early relational wounds. A trauma-informed lens also highlights the importance of co-regulation, which can still occur online but may require more explicit acknowledgment and creative engagement. Psychoanalysis in the digital age must rise to the challenge of making room for trauma, not only as content, but as structure, rhythm, and absence, in order to remain a relevant and reparative practice.

Finally, the digitization of practice opens space for new intersubjective metaphors. What does it mean to "log in" to another person's world? How do we conceptualize the transfer of unconscious material through data streams, images, and bandwidth?

These metaphors are not merely poetic – they shape how therapists attune, interpret, and hold psychic process. As such, a digital psychoanalytic epistemology must evolve alongside the clinical work itself.

This future will belong not to one school of thought, but to those willing to engage complexity, contradiction, and transformation. That, after all, is what psychoanalysis has always asked of us.

Closing Reflections

In closing, this book has charted the complex terrain of online psychodynamic psychotherapy, a landscape shaped by urgency, adaptation, resistance, and creativity. What began as a response to global disruption has become a site of innovation and theoretical development. Far from signaling the dilution of analytic depth, the online medium has revealed new layers of meaning, new modes of presence, and new challenges for the therapeutic relationship.

The digital space does not render the unconscious irrelevant; on the contrary, it reconfigures how the unconscious is expressed, enacted, and interpreted. Transference lives on, shaped by latency, screen imagery, and the paradoxical intimacy of disembodied connection. The therapist's presence, once grounded in physical space, now arises through voice, rhythm, attunement, and the careful construction of digital holding. These developments do not betray psychoanalytic principles; they exemplify their adaptive vitality. Rather than being tied to a fixed physical context, the unconscious proves remarkably fluid, emerging through glitches, silences, digital rituals, and the altered temporality of virtual exchange. The core analytic capacities – listening, containing, interpreting – remain intact, even as they find new forms in the screen-mediated encounter. What changes is not the aim of psychoanalysis, but the frame in which it unfolds, a shift that invites ongoing creativity and theoretical renewal.

At the same time, this evolution is not without cost. The loss of embodied co-presence raises important questions about the limits of empathy, containment, and repair. The risk of mis-attunement, fragmentation, and technological overreach is real. But so too is the opportunity: To reach across distance, to innovate responsibly, and to make psychoanalytic therapy accessible to new populations, new languages, and new forms of psychic life.

Ultimately, online psychodynamic psychotherapy challenges us to return to first principles – not to preserve them in amber, but to re-animate them in contemporary form. This demands humility, creativity, and ethical rigor. It demands that we listen not only to our patients but also to the changing world in which therapy takes place.

In doing so, we honor the deepest values of psychoanalysis: Presence, transformation, and the enduring human search for meaning in the face of uncertainty.

This transformation also compels us to revisit the concept of analytic neutrality. In online spaces, where the therapist's home or facial expressions may be more visible, neutrality becomes a relational, negotiated stance rather than a fixed position. Patients may inquire about the therapist's space, household interruptions, or even internet quality – all of which reconfigure the transference and test the therapist's symbolic position. The task is not to erase these factors but to metabolize them within the analytic process, using curiosity and meaning-making rather than defensiveness or denial. What neutrality comes to mean in this context is a disciplined openness, a willingness to receive projections and explore their meaning, even when triggered by seemingly mundane elements like a background painting or a momentary glitch. This reframing calls on therapists to hold complexity without retreating into idealized detachment, demonstrating that neutrality is not about invisibility, but about reverent responsiveness within a bounded frame.

There is also a growing call for psychoanalytic communities to archive and study their experiences of the digital shift. Case reports, supervision notes, patient reflections, and longitudinal data will help future generations understand the texture of this transition. As digital natives enter training programs, they will bring new assumptions, vocabularies, and modes of embodiment that may further stretch classical models. The psychoanalytic "canon" may expand to include writings on interface, latency, digital affect, and virtual co-presence, concepts that were once peripheral but are now central to practice. This evolving body of knowledge offers not only clinical guidance, but also historical insight into how a traditionally inward-facing discipline responded to a moment of global rupture and technological acceleration. Documenting this shift is not merely a matter of academic interest; it is a form of institutional memory, allowing us to track how psychoanalysis sustains its relevance by remaining open to transformation.

As we close, we must acknowledge that the psychoanalytic project, so often portrayed as slow, interior, and retrospective, has adapted with remarkable speed. The field's responsiveness to digital practice is not a break from tradition, but a testament to its generativity. At its heart, psychoanalysis remains an encounter between subjectivities, a site where pain becomes language, and where silence may still speak. Whether face-to-face or screen-to-screen, this task continues.

References

Agar, G. (2020). The clinic offers no advantage over the screen, for relationship is everything. In H. Weinberg & A. Rolnick (Eds.), *Theory and practice of online therapy: Internet-delivered interventions for individuals, families, groups, and organizations* (pp. 66–78). Routledge.

APA [American Psychological Association]. (2023). Psychologists reaching their limits as patients present with worsening symptoms year after year: 2023 Practitioner Pulse Survey. Retrieved from htps://www.apa.org/pubs/reports/pracctitioner/2023-psychologist-reach-limits.

APsA [American Psychoanalytic Association]. (n.d.). Retrieved 23 December 2024 from https://apsa.org/about-psychoanalysis/psychoanalytic-theory-approaches/#toggle-id-1.

Andersson, G. (2016). Internet-delivered psychological treatments. *Annual Review of Clinical Psychology.* 12: 157–179. doi:10.1146/annurev-clinpsy-021815-093006.

Andersson, G. (2018). Internet interventions: Past, present and future. *Internet Interventions* 12: 181–188. doi:10.1016/j.invent.2018.03.008.

Andrews, K., Ross, D., & Maroney, T.L. (2024). Online group psychotherapy: A systematic review. *Community Mental Health Journal.* doi:10.1007/s10597-024-01304-4.

Anzieu, D. (1985). *The skin ego.* (Trans. C. Turner, 1989). Yale University Press.

Aron, L. (1996). *A meeting of minds: Mutuality in psychoanalysis.* Analytic Press.

Avula, V.C.R., & Amalakanti, S. (2025). Artificial intelligence trends in psychiatry, present trends and challenges: an updated review. *International Journal of Neuropsychopharmacology,* 28 (1): i213. doi:10.1093/ijnp/pyae059.373.

Backhaus, A., Agha, Z., Maglione, M.L., Repp, A., Ross, B., Zuest, D., Rice-Thorp, N.M., Lohr, J., & Thorp, S.R. (2012). Videoconferencing psychotherapy: A systematic review. *Psychological Services*, 9 (2): 111–131. doi:10.1037/a0027924.

Bagnini, C. (2015). Technology stirred projective processes in couple tele therapy. In: J.S. Scharff (Ed.), *Psychoanalysis Online* (pp. 186–195). Routledge.

Bar, V. (2023). Me and my "Otherness". Or: Who is the Other on the screen who looks exactly like me? In H. Weinberg, A. Rolnick, & A. Leighton (Eds.), *Advances in online therapy: Emergence of a new paradigm* (pp. 73–83). Routledge.

Barak, A., Grohol, J.M., & Patlamazoglou, L.M. (2004). A comprehensive review and a meta-analysis of the effectiveness of internet-based psychotherapeutic interventions. *Journal of Technology in Human Services*, 22: 37–55.

Beebe, B., & Lachmann, F. (2002). *Infant research and adult treatment: Co-constructing interactions.* Analytic Press.

Benjamin, J. (1995). *Like subjects, love objects.* Yale University Press.

Benjamin, J. (2004). Beyond doer and done to: An intersubjective view of thirdness. *The Psychoanalytic Quarterly*, 73 (1): 5–46.

Berryhill, M.B., Culmer, N., Williams, N., Halli-Tierney, A., Betancourt, A., Roberts, H., & King, M. (2019). Videoconferencing psychotherapy and depression: A systematic review. *Telemedicine and e-Health*, 25 (6): 435–446. doi:10.1089/tmj.2018.0058.

Bleger, J. (1967/2018). Psychoanalysis of the psychoanalytic setting. In A. Harris & I. Tylim (Eds.), *Reconsidering the moveable frame in psychoanalysis. Its function and structure in contemporary psychoanalytic theory* (p. 22). Routledge.

Braude, G., Mohi, S., Quinlan, E., Shoullis, A., & Collison, J. (2023). A change in frame and countertransference experiences: Transitioning from face-to-face to telepsychotherapy. *Counselling & Psychotherapy Research*, 23 (4): 1063–1071. doi:10.1002/capr.12612.

Burlingame, G.M., Fuhriman, A., & Johnson, J.E. (2001). Cohesion in group psychotherapy. *Psychotherapy: Theory, Research, Practice, Training*, 38 (4): 373–379.

Burlingame, G.M., McClendon, D.T., & Yang, C. (2018). Cohesion in group therapy: A meta-analysis. *Psychotherapy*, 55 (4): 384–398. doi:10.1037/pst0000173.

Callan, J.E., Maheu, M.M., & Bucky, S.F. (2017). Crisis in the behavioral health classroom: Enhancing knowledge, skills, and attitudes in telehealth training. In M.M. Maheu, K. Drude, & S. Wright (Eds.), *Career paths in telemental health* (pp. 63–80). Springer.

Carlino, R. (2011). *Distance psychoanalysis: The theory and practice of using communication technology in the clinic*. Karnac.

Chavooshi, B., Mohammadkhani, P., & Dolatshahi, B. (2016). A randomized double-blind controlled trial comparing Davanloo intensive short-term dynamic psychotherapy as internet-delivered vs treatment as usual for medically unexplained pain: A 6-month pilot study. *Psychosomatics*, 57 (3): 292–300. doi:10.1016/j.psym.2016.01.001.

Dehbozorgi, R., Zangeneh, S., Khooshab, E., Nia, D.H., Hanif, H.R., Samian, P., Yousefi, M., Hashemi, F.H., Vakili, M., Jamalimoghadam, N., & Lohrasebi, F. (2025). The application of artificial intelligence in the field of mental health: A systematic review. *BMC Psychiatry*, 25: 132. doi:10.1186/s12888-025-06483-2.

Derrig-Palumbo, K., & Zeine, F. (2005). *Online therapy: A therapist's guide to expanding your practice*. Norton.

Dolev-Amit et al. 2020 has been added to Ch 4 as part of the query process

Dolev-Amit, T., Leibovich, L., & Zilcha-Mano, S. (2020). Repairing alliance ruptures using supportive techniques in telepsychotherapy during the COVID-19 pandemic. *Counselling Psychology Quarterly*, 34 (3–4): 485–498. doi:10.1080/09515070.2020.1777089.

Dudai, O., & Metzl, E. (2024). I can hide if I want to: The function of the screen in Zoom psychotherapy. *Psychoanalysis, Culture & Society*. doi:10.1057/s41282-024-00484-y.

Eichenberger, A., & Boswell, N. (2024). Transference in teletherapy: A case discussion. *The American Journal of Psychiatry Residents' Journal*, 19 (4): 18–19. doi:10.1176/appi.ajp-rj.2024.190407.

Eubanks, C.F., Muran, J.C., & Safran, J.D. (2018). Alliance rupture repair: A meta-analysis. *Psychotherapy*, 55 (4): 508–519. doi: doi:10.1037/pst0000185.

Fairbairn, W. (1953). *Psychoanalytic studies of the personality*. Tavistock Publications.

Fernandez, E., Woldgabreal, Y., Day, A., Pham, T., Gleich, B., & Aboujaoude, E. (2021). Live psychotherapy by video versus in-person: A meta-analysis of efficacy and its relationship to types and targets of treatment. *Clinical Psychology & Psychotherapy*, 28 (6): 1535–1549. doi:10.1002/cpp.2594.

Flückiger, C., Rubel, J., Del Re, A.C., Horvath, A.O., Wampold, B.E., Crits-Christoph, P., Atzil-Slonim, D., Compare, A., Falkenstrom, F., Ekeblad, A., Errazuriz, P., Fisher, H., Hofart, A., Huppert, J.D., Kivity, Y., Kumar, M., Lutz, W., Muran, J.C., & Strunk, D.R., …, &Barber, J. (2020). The reciprocal relationship between alliance and early treatment symptoms: A two-stage individual participant data meta-analysis. *Journal of Consulting and Clinical Psychology*, 88 (9): 829–843. doi:10.1037/cou0000424.

Foulkes, S.H. (1975). *Group analytic psychotherapy: Method and principles.* Gordon andBreach (reissued Karnac, 1986 and 1991).

Freud, A. (1936). *The ego and the mechanisms of defense.* The writings of Anna Freud, Volume 2. International Universities Press (published 1967–1983).

Freud, S. (1895). *Studies on hysteria* (with J. Breuer). The Standard Edition of the Complete Psychological Works of Sigmund Freud, Volume 2. Hogarth Press (published 1953–1974).

Freud, S. (1913). *On beginning the treatment (further recommendations on the technique of psychoanalysis I)*. The Standard Edition of the Complete Psychological Works of Sigmund Freud, Volume 12. Hogarth Press (published 1953–1974).

Freud, S. (1915). *The unconscious* (pp. 159–204). The Standard Edition of the Complete Psychological Works of Sigmund Freud, Volume 14. Hogarth Press (published 1953–1974).

Freud, S. (1923). *The ego and the id.* The Standard Edition of the Complete Psychological Works of Sigmund Freud, Volume 12. Hogarth Press.

Friedman, R. (2023) Group analytic therapy and the online groups: Some principles of the group analytic approach to online group therapy. In H. Weinberg, A. Rolnick, & A. Leighton (Eds.), *The virtual group therapy circle: Advances in online group theory and practice* (pp. 101–111). Routledge.

Gabbard, G.O. (1994). Psychotherapists who transgress sexual boundaries with patients. *Bulletin of the Menninger Clinic*, 58 (1): 124–135.

Gabbard, G.O. (2010). *Long-term psychodynamic psychotherapy: A basic text.* American Psychiatric Publishing.

Geller, S.M. (2023). Being present and together while apart: Therapeutic presence in telepsychotherapy. In H. Weinberg, A. Rolnick, & A. Leighton (Eds.), *Advances in online therapy: Emergence of a new paradigm* (pp. 21–34). Routledge. doi:10.4324/9781003205029.

Geller, S.M., & Greenberg, L.S. (2012). *Therapeutic presence: A mindful approach to effective therapy.* APA Publications.

Geltner, P. (2006). The concept of objective countertransference and its role in a two-person psychology. *American Journal of Psychoanalysis*, 66: 25–42. doi:10.1007/s11231-005-9001-3.

Giovanetti, A.K., Punt, S.E.W., Nelson, E., & Ilardi, S.S. (2022). Teletherapy versus in-person psychotherapy for depression: A meta-analysis of randomized controlled trials. *Telemedicine and e-Health*, 28 (8): 1077–1089. doi:10.1089/tmj.2021.0294.

Glueckauf, R.L., Maheu, M.M., Drude, K.P., Wells, B.A., Wang, Y., Gustafson, D.J., & Nelson, E.-L. (2018). Survey of psychologists' telebehavioral health practices: Technology use, ethical issues, and training needs. *Professional Psychology Resource Practice*, 49: 205–219. doi:10.1037/pro0000188.

Godleski, L., Darkins, A., Peters, J. (2012). Outcomes of 98,609 U.S. Department of Veterans Affairs patients enrolled in telemental health services, 2006–2010. *Psychiatric Services*, 63 (4): 383–385. doi:10.1176/appi.ps.201100206.

Gotti, M. (2024). From the gate to the gateway: Psychoanalytic navigations online. *American Journal of Psychoanalysis*, 84: 229–249. doi:10.1057/s11231-024-09446-w.

Greenberg, J., & Mitchell, S. (1983). *Object relations in psychoanalytic theory*. Harvard University Press. doi:10.2307/j.ctvjk2xv6.

Greenwood, H., Krzyzaniak, N., Peiris, R., Clark, J., Scott, A.M., Cardona, M., Griffith, R., & Glasziou, P. (2022). Telehealth versus face-to-face psychotherapy for less common mental health conditions: Systematic review and meta-analysis of randomized controlled trials. *JMIR Mental Health*, 9 (3): e31780. doi:10.2196/31780.

Griffiths, K.M., Farrer, L., & Christie, G. (2010). Effectiveness of online cognitive behavioral therapy in maintaining remission from depression. *Journal of Consulting and Clinical Psychology*, 78: 160–169.

Grossmark, R. (2007). The edge of chaos: Enactment, disruption, and emergence in group psychotherapy. *Psychoanalytic Dialogues*, 17 (4): 479–499.

Haber, Y., Levkovich, I., Hadar-Shoval, D., & Elyoseph, Z. (2024). The artificial third: A broad view of the effects of introducing generative artificial intelligence on psychotherapy. *JMRI Mental Health*, 11: e54781. doi:10.2196/54781.

Haberstroh, S., Barney, L., Foster, N., & Duffey, T. (2014). The ethical and legal practice of online counseling and psychotherapy: A review of mental health professions. *Journal of Technology in Human Services*, 32 (3): 149–157. doi:10.1080/15228835.2013.872074.

Haddouk, L. (2015). Presence at a distance. *Annual Review of Cybertherapy and Telemedicine*, 13: 208–212.

Harris, A. (2005). Transference, countertransference, and the real relationship. In E.S. Person, A.M. Cooper, & G.O. Gabbard (Eds.), *The American psychiatric publishing textbook of psychoanalysis* (pp. 201–216). American Psychiatric Publishing.

Harris, A. & Tylim, I. (2018). Introduction: The frame. In A. Harris & I. Tylim (Eds.), *Reconsidering the moveable frame in psychoanalysis. Its function and structure in contemporary psychoanalytic theory* (pp. 1–11). Routledge.

Hartmann, H. (1958). *Ego psychology and the problem of adaptation.* (Trans. D. Rapaport). International Universities Press. doi:10.1037/13180-000.

Heimann, P. (1950). On counter-transference. *International Journal of Psycho-Analysis*, 31: 81–84.

Hilty, D.M., Ferrer, D.C., Burke Parish, M., Johnston, B., Callahan, E.J., & Yellowlees, P.M. (2013). The effectiveness of telemental health: A 2013 review. *Telemedicine and e-Health*, 19 (6): 444–454. doi:10.1089/tmj.2013.0075.

Hopper, E. (2001). The social unconscious: Theoretical considerations. *Group Analysis*, 34 (1): 9–27.

Hopper, E. (Ed.) (2023). *The social unconscious in persons, groups and societies.* Volume IV. *The tripartite matrix in the developing theory and expanding practice of group analysis.* Routledge.

Hopper, E., & Weinberg, H. (Eds.). (2011). *The social unconscious in persons, groups and societies.* Volume 1. *Mainly Theory.* Karnac.

Hopper, E. & Weinberg, H. (Eds.) (2015). *The social unconscious in persons, groups and societies.* Volume 2. *Mainly foundation matrices.* Karnac.

Hopper, E. & Weinberg, H. (Eds.) (2017). *The social unconscious in persons, groups and societies: Volume 3: The foundation matrix extended and reconfigured.* Karnac.

Horvath, A.O., & Symonds, B.D. (1991). Relation between working alliance and outcome in psychotherapy: A meta-analysis. *Journal of Counseling Psychology*, 38 (2): 139–149.

Humer, E., Schramm, E., Klein, J.P., Härter, M., Hautzinger, M., Pieh, C., & Probst, T. (2021) Effects of alliance ruptures and repairs on outcomes. *Psychotherapy Research*, 31 (8): 977–987.

Keating, B. (2023). Diving into the world of online play therapy. In H. Weinberg, A. Rolnick, & A. Leighton (Eds.), *Advances in online therapy: Emergence of a new paradigm* (pp. 299–307). Routledge.

Kegerreis, S. (2022). The experience of time boundaries in remote working. *British Journal of Psychotherapy*, 38 (4): 754–768. doi:10.1111/bjp.12768.

Kernberg, O.F. (2016). Psychoanalytic theories of personality. In H.S. Friedman & R.C. Silver (Eds.), *Handbook of medical psychology* (pp. 69–82). Springer.

King, V.L., Brooner, R.K., Peirce, J.M., Kolodner, K., & Kidorf, M.S. (2014). A randomized trial of web-based videoconferencing for substance abuse counseling. *Journal of Substance Abuse Treatment*, 46 (1): 36–42.

Kingsley, A., & Henning, J.A. (2015). Online and phone therapy: Challenges and opportunities. *The Journal of Individual Psychology*, 71 (2): 185–194.

Klein, M. (1923). The development of a child. *International Journal of Psycho-Analysis*, 4: 419–474.

Klein, M. (1935). A contribution to the psychogenesis of manic-depressive states. *International Journal of Psycho-Analysis*, 16: 145–174.

Kleinplatz, P.J., Charest, M., Paradis, N., Rosen, L.A., Lawless, S., & Ramsay, T. (2024). Remote versus in-person group therapy for couples distressed by low/no sexual desire/frequency or sexual desire discrepancy: A response to COVID-19. *Journal of Couple & Relationship Therapy*: 1–21. doi:10.1080/15332691.2024.2343730.

Kohut, H. (1971). *The Analysis of the Self*. University of Chicago Press.

Kranzberg, M. (1986). Technology and history: Kranzberg's laws. *Technology and Culture*, 27 (3): 544–560.

Lange, A., Rietdijk, D., Hudcovicova, M., van de Ven, J.P., Schrieken, B., Emmelkamp, P.M.G. (2003). Interapy: A controlled randomized trial of the standardized treatment of posttraumatic stress through the internet. *Journal of Consulting and Clinical Psychology*, 71 (5): 901–909.

Langs, R. (1998). *Ground rules in psychotherapy and counseling*. Karnac.

Larsson, M.H., Falkenström, F., Andersson, G., & Holmqvist, R. (2018). Alliance ruptures and repairs in psychotherapy in primary care. *Psychotherapy Research*, 28 (1): 123–136. doi:10.1080/10503307.2016.1174345.

Lemma, A. (2017). *The digital age on the couch*. Routledge.

Lemma, A. (2020). *Psychoanalysis in times of technoculture*. Routledge.

Marmarosh, C., Robelo, A., Solorio, A., & Xing, F. (2023). Miles away: Alliance and cohesion in online group therapy. In H. Weinberg, A. Rolnick, & A. Leighton (Eds.), *The virtual group therapy circle: Advances in online group theory and practice* (pp. 40–51). Routledge.

Matheson, C., & Kegerreis, S. (2023). "The genie's out of the bottle": The impact of working online with individual psychodynamic psychotherapy for therapists and clients, and its lessons for psychodynamic training. *British Journal of Psychotherapy*, 39 (3): 573–591. doi:10.1111/bjp.12853.

Messina, I., & Loffler-Stastka, H. (2021). Psychotherapists' perception of their clinical skills and in-session feelings in live therapy versus online therapy during the COVID-19 pandemic: a pilot study. *Research in Psychotherapy*, 24 (1): 514. doi:10.4081/ripppo.2021.514.

Miller-Bottome, M., Talia, A., Eubanks, C.F., Safran, J.D., & Muran, J. C. (2019). Secure in-session attachment predicts rupture resolution: Negotiating a secure base. *Psychoanalytic Psychology*, 36 (2): 132–138. doi:10.1037/pap0000232.

Mitchell, S.A. (1988). *Relational concepts in psychoanalysis.* Harvard University Press.

Modell, A.H. (1989). The psychoanalytic setting as a container of multiple levels of reality: A Perspective on the theory of psychoanalytic treatment. *Psychoanalytic Inquiry*, 9: 67–87.

Muran, C.J., Eubanks, C.F., & Samstag, L.W. (2022). Introduction: Rupture in a wicked and wonderful world. In C.F. Eubanks, L.W. Samstag, & J.C. Muran (Eds.), *Rupture and repair in psychotherapy* (pp. 4–20). APA Publications.

Myers, K., Nelson, E., Rabinowitz, T., Hilty, D., Baker, D., Smucker Barnwell, S., Boyce, G., Bufka, L.F., Cain, S., Chui, L., Comer, J.S., Cradock, C., Goldstein, F., Johnston, B., Krupinski, E., Lo, K., Luxton, D.D., McSwain, S.D., McWilliams, J., ..., & Bernard, J. (2017). American Telemedicine Association practice guidelines for telemental health with children and adolescents. *Telemedicine and e-Health*, 23 (10): 779–804. doi:10.1089/tmj.2017.0177.

Ogden, P., & Goldstein, B. (2020). Sensorimotor psychotherapy from a distance: Engaging the body, creating presence, and building relationship in videoconferencing. In H. Weinberg & A. Rolnick (Eds.), *Theory and practice of online therapy: Internet-delivered interventions for individuals, groups, families, and organizations* (pp. 63–81). Routledge.

Ogden, T.H. (1997). Reverie and interpretation. *The Psychoanalytic Quarterly*, 66 (4): 567–595.

Ogden, T.H, (2004). The analytic third: Implications for psychoanalytic theory and technique. *The Psychoanalytic Quarterly*, 73 (1): 167–195.

Possati, L.M. (2020). Algorithmic unconscious: Why psychoanalysis helps in understanding AI. *Palgrave Communications*, 6: 70. doi:10.1057/s41599-020-0445-0.

Psychoanalytic Perspectives. (2017). Special issue, 14 (2). doi:10.1080/1551806X.2017.1304111.

Rasmussen, B., Perry, R., Hickey, M., Hua, X., Wong, Z.W., Guy, L., Hitch, D., Hiscock, H., Dalziel, K., Winter, N., & Maier, A.B. (2022). Patient preferences using telehealth during the COVID-19 pandemic in four Victorian tertiary hospital services. *Internal Medicine Journal*, 52 (5): 763–769. doi:10.1111/imj.15726.

Russell, G.I. (2015). *Screen relations.* Karnac.

Rutan, J.S., Stone, W.N., & Shay, J.J. (2014). *Psychodynamic group psychotherapy* (5th ed.). Guilford Press.

Safran, J.D., & Muran, J.C. (2000). *Negotiating the therapeutic alliance: A relational treatment guide.* Guilford Press.

Sampaio, M., Navarro Haro, M.V., De Sousa, B., Vieira Melo, W., & Hoffman, H.G. (2021). Therapists make the switch to telepsychology to safely continue treating their patients during the COVID-19 pandemic. Virtual reality telepsychology may be next. *Frontiers in Virtual Reality*, 1: 576421. doi:10.3389/frvir.2020.576421.

Scharff, J.S. (Ed.). (2013). *Psychoanalysis online: Mental health, teletherapy and training*. Karnac.

Scharff, J.S. (Ed.). (2015). *Psychoanalysis online 2: Impact of technology on development, training, and therapy.* Karnac.

Scharff, J.S., (Ed.). (2017). *Psychoanalysis Online 3: The teleanalytic setting*. Karnac.

Scharff, J.S. (Ed.). (2018). *Psychoanalysis Online 4: Teleanalytic practice, teaching, and clinical research*. Routledge.

Scharff, J.S., & Scharff, D.E. (2000). Object relations couple therapy. *American journal of psychotherapy, 51* (2): 141–173.

Shedler, J. (2010). The efficacy of psychodynamic psychotherapy. *American Psychologist*, 65 (2): 98–109.

Shoullis, A., Mohi, S., Quinlan, E., Collison, J., & Braude, G. (2023). Change to the therapeutic frame: Exploring the therapeutic alliance when transitioning from face-to-face therapy to videoconferencing. *International Journal for the Advancement of Counselling*, 45: 458–474. doi:10.1007/s10447-023-09516-1.

Simpson, S.G., & Reid, C.L. (2014). Therapeutic alliance in videoconferencing psychotherapy: A review. *Australian Journal of Rural Health*, 22 (6): 280–299. doi:10.1111/ajr.12149.

Singh, O.P. (2024). Artificial intelligence and psychoanalysis: A new concept of research methodology. *NPRC Journal of Multidisciplinary Research*, 1: 19–27. doi:10.3126/nprcjmr.v1i1.69012.

Slone, N.C., Reese, R.J., & McClellan, M.J. (2012). Telepsychology outcome research with children and adolescents: A review of the literature. *Psychological Services*, 9 (3): 272–292. doi:10.1037/a0027607.

Stern, D.N. (1985). *The interpersonal world of the infant*. Basic Books.

Sucala, M., Schnur, J.B., Constantino, M.J., Miller, S.J., Brackman, E.H., & Montgomery, G.H. (2012). The therapeutic relationship in e-therapy for mental health: A systematic review. *Journal of Medical Internet Research*, 14 (4): 175–187. doi:10.2196/jmir.2084.

Triest, Y. (2011, July 2). Between "law" and "lap" – Reflections on border patrol and issues of containment. Hebrew Psychology. Retrieved 27 February 2022 from https://www.hebpsy.net/articles.asp?id=2622.

Tronick, E.Z., Als, H., Adamson, L., Wise, S., & Brazelton, T.B. (1978). The infant's response to entrapment between contradictory messages in face-to-face interaction. *Journal of the American Academy of Child Psychiatry*, 17 (1): 1–13.

Trop, G. (2021). Virtual containments: Abstinence and the frame in online psychoanalysis . *Psychoanalytic Dialogues*, 31 (3): 321–337.

Trub, L.R. (2024). The elephant in the zoom: Will psychoanalysis survive the screen? *American Journal of Psychoanalysis*, 84 (2): 203–228. doi:10.1057/s11231-024-09457-7.

Turgoose, D., Ashwick, R., & Murphy, D. (2018). Systematic review of lessons learned from delivering tele-therapy to veterans with post-traumatic stress disorder. *Journal of Telemedicine and Telecare*, 24 (9): 575–585. doi:10.1177/1357633X17730443.

Turkle, S. (2005). *The second self: Computers and the human spirit*(Twentieth Anniversary Edition). MIT Press. doi: doi:10.7551/mitpress/6115.001.0001.

Turkle, S. (2011). *Alone together: Why we expect more from technology and less from each other*. Basic Books.

Turkle, S., Essig, T., & Russell, G.I. (2017). Afterword: Reclaiming psychoanalysis: Sherry Turkle in conversation with the editors. *Psychoanalytic Perspectives*, 14 (2): 237–248.

Varker, T., Brand, R.M., Ward, J., Terhaag, S., & Phelps, A. (2019). Efficacy of synchronous telepsychology interventions for people with anxiety, depression, posttraumatic stress disorder, and adjustment disorder: A rapid evidence assessment. *Psychological Services*, 16 (4): 621–635. doi:10.1037/ser0000239.

Weinberg, H. (2014). *The paradox of internet groups: Alone in the presence of virtual others*. Karnac.

Weinberg, H. (2020a). Online group psychotherapy: Challenges and possibilities during COVID-19 – A practice review. *Group Dynamics: Theory, Research, and Practice*, 24 (3): 201–211. doi:10.1037/gdn0000140.

Weinberg, H. (2020b). Online group therapy – In search of a new theory? In H. Weinberg & A. Rolnick (Eds.), *Theory and practice of online therapy: Internet-delivered interventions for individuals, families, groups, and organizations* (pp. 172–184). Routledge.

Weinberg, H. (2021). Obstacles, challenges, and benefits of online group psychotherapy. *American Journal of Psychotherapy*, 74 (2): 83–88. doi:10.1176/appi.psychotherapy.20200034.

Weinberg, H. (2025). Resistances to online group analysis – Is there anything new under the sun? *Group Analysis*, 58 (1): 49–60. doi:10.1177/05333164251315825.

Weinberg, H., & Rolnick, A. (Eds.). (2020). *Theory and practice of online therapy.* Routledge.

Weinberg, H., Rolnick A., & Leighton, A. (Eds.). (2023). *Advances in online therapy: Emergence of a new paradigm.* Routledge.

Weiner, I.B., & Bornstein, R.F. (2009). *Principles of psychotherapy: Promoting evidence-based psychodynamic practice* (3rd ed.). Wiley.

Winnicott, D.W. (1953). Transitional objects and transitional phenomena. *International Journal of Psychoanalysis*, 34: 89–97.

Winnicott, D.W. (1955). Metapsychological and clinical aspects of regression within the psycho-analytical set-up. *International Journal of Psychoanalysis*, 36: 16–26.

Winnicott, D.W. (1960). The theory of the parent-infant relationship. *International Journal of Psychoanalysis*, 41: 585–595.

Winnicott, D.W. (1965). *The maturational process and the facilitating environment.* Hogarth Press.

Zeavin, H. (2021). *The distance cure: A history of teletherapy.* MIT Press. doi: doi:10.7551/mitpress/12823.001.0001.

Zimmerman, M., Ward, M., D'Avanzato, C., & Tirpak, J.W. (2021). Telehealth treatment of patients with borderline personality disorder in a partial hospital setting during the COVID-19 pandemic: Comparative safety, patient satisfaction, and effectiveness of in-person treatment. *Journal of Personality Disorders*, 36 (3): 277–295. doi:10.1521/pedi_2021_35_539.

Index

Made in the USA
Monee, IL
13 September 2026

62978586R00085